THE BENEFITS OF NOT GROWING OLDER

Unlocking the Secrets to a Vibrant Life

"The Benefits of Not Growing Older" provides a roadmap for aging with grace, purpose, and vitality, offering a vision of growth and renewal.

James Mason

TABLE OF CONTENT

12.3 Embracing Change and Finding Joy in Every Stage

INTRODUCTION

Welcome to the journey that questions social standards, goes against the grain, and discovers the amazing advantages of delaying aging. This investigation aims to reveal the unrealized potential, undiscovered pleasures, and life-changing opportunities that exist outside the confines of time in a society that is preoccupied with the inevitable passage of time.

Imagine living a life in which time does not rob you of your energy but instead presents you with a constant stream of fresh experiences and chances. Despite popular belief, there are numerous benefits to adopting a mindset that challenges the traditional aging paradigm, including mental, emotional, spiritual, and physical benefits.

We will traverse the domains of health and wellbeing as we set out on this quest for agelessness, refuting the idea that aging is an irreversible decline. We'll dive in

CHAPTER ONE

In a world where age often comes with a set of predefined expectations, defying age stereotypes becomes a rebellious declaration of individuality. It's an exhilarating act of refusing to conform to society's narrow views on growing older, and instead, embracing the freedom to redefine what it means to age.

Imagine a world where wrinkles are not battle scars but intricate maps of a life well-lived, where gray hair is not a sign of fading but a crown of wisdom proudly worn. Defying age stereotypes is an invitation to challenge conventional standards of beauty and embrace the unique allure that comes with the passage of time.

This rebellion against the ticking clock extends beyond appearance. It's about rewriting life's script, tearing up the expected timeline, and reveling in the freedom to pursue passions, dreams, and new adventures at any age. Whether it's breaking athletic records in the golden years or discovering hidden talents later in life, defying age stereotypes is a celebration of resilience and untapped potential.

Cognitive empowerment becomes a weapon in this rebellion—where lifelong learning and technological prowess defy the notion that minds inevitably stagnate with age. It's about proving that the brain is a dynamic, ever-adapting organ capable of continuous growth and innovation.

Physical resilience takes center stage, not as a fight against aging, but as a dance with vitality. Exercise becomes a celebration of what the body can achieve, and nutrition is a way to fuel the energy needed to conquer new challenges, defying the physical limitations society may impose.

The rebellion extends to mindset, where positivity becomes a shield against self-imposed limitations. Ageism is challenged, dismantled, and replaced with a society that values the richness of experience, regardless of the number of years lived.

Living with purpose turns into the rebellion's motto, proclaiming that age is no barrier to contributing to the world and that life's changes are chances for personal development. Making a lasting impression becomes the ultimate way to reject the idea that growing older equals becoming less visible.

THE FASCINATION WITH YOUTHFULNESS

The obsession with youthfulness in a world where the idea of perpetual youth captivates people extends beyond the need to rewind time to include a search to discover the secrets of vitality, energy, and limitless potential that seem to go hand in hand with the exuberance of youth.

Imagine the curiosity as a force that draws us in, like a moth to a flame, to the exuberance of youth. It's more than simply glowing skin and flawless smiles—it's a heady mix of perseverance, curiosity, and an unquenchable need for new experiences. Being youthful turns into a mentality—a concoction that transcends the limitations of traditional age.

This is not only about aesthetics on the surface. It's about having an insatiable curiosity, having the guts to take chances, and having unwavering faith.

CHAPTER TWO

UNDERSTANDING THE AGING PROCESS

While aging is sometimes depicted as an unavoidable process, in reality, it develops like a symphony, with each note playing a vital role in the creation of our life as a whole. Instead of viewing aging as a one-dimensional path towards degeneration, let's embark on an expedition to uncover the subtleties of this symphony and understand it as a complex and delicately nuanced composition.

Imagine the aging process as a well-tuned orchestra, where each instrument is a part of our mental, emotional, and physical selves. The woodwinds expressing the subtle changes in our cognitive capacities, the brass signifying the power and resilience that comes with experience, and the strings representing the physical changes—wrinkles carved like musical notes—all combine to create a tune that resonates with the richness of a life properly lived.

Time is the conductor of this symphony, arranging the steps and setting the pace for aging. Time ceases to be an enemy to be overcome and instead turns into a master weaver, tying together the strands of our life to create a masterpiece of development, insight, and changing beauty.

Knowing how aging occurs invites one to investigate the science underlying it and appreciate the molecular dance that occurs inside our bodies. It's an exploration of the worlds of environment, lifestyle, and heredity, where each element plays a part in the graceful dance of aging.

However, this symphony's emotional resonance is just as important to its beauty as its scientific notation. It's about accepting the lines of laughing that convey happy tales, realizing the realizing that age is a highly personal and distinct composition, and that events mold our crescendos and diminuendos.

Therefore, rather than viewing the aging process as a terrifying necessity, let's view it as a chance to comprehend the complex song of time. Like any masterpiece, the symphony of aging may reveal itself to be more profound and resonant with each passing movement as we learn to interpret it.

BIOLOGICAL ASPECTS OF AGING

Our bodies are amazing time machines that are always evolving and adjusting. However, as those years pass, what happens? That's the ageing domain, an intricate dance of biological processes with a few unexpected twists.

Visualize your cells as miniature factories with the Cellular Symphony. Their machinery is subject to wear and tear with time, much like that of an ancient workplace. Proteins can misfold, which causes problems with smooth operation, and DNA can copy itself a little less perfectly.

Twists in Telomeres: Visualize your telomeres as the protecting caps on your DNA. They get shorter with every cell division, until finally they send out a "stop work" signal. However, some people's telomeres tick more slowly than others, so it's not just a straightforward countdown!

Free Radical Rebels: These vivacious molecules resemble microscopic miscreants, bouncing around and destroying essential elements like proteins. as well as DNA. Their natural adversaries are antioxidants, although maintaining equilibrium is essential.

Genes of Longevity: A few fortunate people are born with genes that appear to increase their resistance to aging. Don't worry, though; lifestyle and surroundings also matter a lot! Consider healthy practices as your own anti-aging toolset, including exercise, a balanced diet, and stress reduction.

PSYCHOLOGICAL PERSPECTIVES ON AGING

Aging, which is frequently viewed through the prism of biology, is also a psychological journey, a fascinating investigation of the mind's resilience, adaptability, and capacity for growth. Let's take an interesting look at the psychological viewpoints that depict aging as a dawning of wisdom and self-awareness, rather than as a sunset.

1. **Good Psychology:** Bringing Light to the Golden Years

Positive psychology turns attention away from the difficulties of aging and toward the opportunities it offers. This viewpoint promotes resilience and a sense of fulfillment by encouraging people to embrace the positive aspects of their lives rather than focusing on their limitations. Growing older provides an opportunity for introspection and the development of thankfulness, which enhances mental health.

2. **Life Span Development:** The Constantly Developing Story Understanding aging via a life span Using a development lens, we can recognize how growth continues throughout life. It recognizes that growth is a continuous process that presents different chances and difficulties at every stage of life. Growing older turns aging into a story of adaptability and ongoing change that always leads to a better understanding of oneself.

3. **Erikson's Psychosocial Stages:** Making Your Way Through

According to Erikson's theory of psychosocial development, aging is viewed as a sequence of stages, each of which has unique psychosocial difficulties. This view offers a road map for negotiating the psychological landscape of aging, from the search for identity in youth to the search for integrity and significance in older years. It suggests that later life is a chance for deep self-discovery rather than a time of stagnation.

4. **Wisdom and Cognitive Aging** ;Years Beyond

While age may cause changes in cognitive capacities, psychological research shows that some areas of cognition, such wisdom and emotional intelligence, tend to get better with age. Senior citizens frequently exhibit enhanced emotional control, a deep comprehension of complicated situations, and a plethora of life experience. Reaching the highest level of mental and emotional health is the goal of aging.

5. Redefining Social Priorities through Socioemotional Selectivity Theory

People's priorities change in social circles as they get older. According to the socioemotional selectivity theory, relationships that are emotionally important are prioritized by older adults over those that are based solely on social utility. This viewpoint emphasizes the value of quality over quantity in interpersonal relationships, transforming the aging process into a time of rich social connections.

6. **Resilience and Coping Mechanisms:** Adapting to Difficulties Psychological viewpoints on aging highlight the incredible fortitude people display when confronted with obstacles in life. By using healthy coping mechanisms, people can age gracefully and adaptably through all of life's ups and downs. Growing older becomes a symbol of the human spirit's ability to persevere, adapt, and develop.

The Core: An Emotional Tapestry

By investigating psychological viewpoints on aging, we reveal a mosaic of fortitude, development, and knowledge. Aging is not a story of decline, but rather a fascinating psychological journey that reveals the complexity and depth of the human psyche. The journey's core is not only comprehending how the mind reacts to time, but also appreciating the psychological tapestry that is constructed throughout time and exposing the ultimate masterpiece that eventually appears

CHAPTER THREE

THE SURPRISING HEALTH ADVANTAGES

There are several unexpected benefits to health that go beyond the traditional domains and are frequently seen through the prisms of diet and exercise. Let's explore the lesser-known but incredibly fascinating facets of wellbeing and the unanticipated advantages that lead to a whole and satisfying existence.

1. Laughing Therapy: The Happy Cure

Laughter is a healing elixir for the body and mind, and is frequently considered the best medicine. It is more than just entertainment. Laughing has been scientifically shown to lower stress hormones, boost immunity, and release endorphins. It is a natural remedy for general well-being. Thus, remember that the next time you find yourself laughing heartily, you are doing more for your health than merely enjoying yourself.

2. Cozy Culture: The Influence of Physical Contact

Cuddling and physical touch have significant health benefits that go beyond romantic gestures. Releasing oxytocin, also known as the "love hormone," has several health benefits, including lowering stress and anxiety and strengthening the immune system. Whether with friends, family, or pets, creating a culture of cuddling turns into an unexpected yet enjoyable way to promote mental and physical well-being.

3. Chocolate Delight: Sweet Delights for the Sensational Heart

Snacking on a dark chocolate square is not only a sinful pleasure but also a heart-healthy treat. Dark chocolate, which is high in antioxidants, has been connected to lowered blood pressure, better mood, and improved cardiovascular health. Thus, remember that the next time you indulge in that rich chocolate, you're doing more for your heart than just pampering your taste senses.

4. Harmonizing Through Music Medicine The body and the soul

Music is more than just entertainment; it's a potent kind of soul therapy. A suitable melody can be a tonic for overall well-being, as it has been scientifically shown to lower stress, improve mood, and even improve cognitive performance. Adding music to your daily routine, whether it be with calming melodies or energetic beats, is an unexpected but powerful remedy for living a happier, healthier life.

5. Green Therapy: The Restorative Power of Nature

Time spent in nature, sometimes called "green therapy," is more than just appreciating beautiful scenery. Stress reduction, mood enhancement, and increased mental health have all been linked to spending time in natural settings. Surprising health benefits from nature's therapeutic touch serve as a reminder to get outside and rediscover the renewing power of the wonderful outdoors.

6. Random Deeds of Goodwill: The Snowball Effect

Random acts of kindness have a surprise health benefit for the giver in addition to making others feel good. According to scientific research, deeds of kindness cause endorphins to be released, which enhances happiness and well-being. Kindness has a beneficial ripple effect that lasts beyond the present situation and improves one's physical and emotional well-being.

The Harmonious Well-Being: Accepting the Unexpected

Accepting these unexpected health benefits adds some joy to the traditional route on the way to well-being. A wellness symphony that transcends expectations is created by laughter, cuddles, chocolate, music, nature, and kindness. It serves as a reminder that there are many different and enjoyable ways to achieve excellent health. life of its own. So let's embrace the unexpected and discover happiness and contentment in the unexpected nooks and crannies of our daily lives.

MAINTAINING PHYSICAL VITALITY

Physical vitality is essential for living a full and active life. Setting our physical health as a top priority becomes increasingly important as we manage the pressures of modern life. Join us as we examine the fundamental ideas and unexpected tactics for preserving physical vitality, making sure that our bodies stay strong, vivacious, and prepared to take on all that life has to offer.

1. Magic of Movement: The Dancing of Well-Being

The key to physical vitality is in movement. Moving every day becomes more than just an organized exercise program; it becomes a joyful celebration of your health. Find things that make you happy and keep your body moving, whether it's a vigorous walk, a dance class, or a stroll through the outdoors. The beginning of the well-being dance is the straightforward action of moving forward one foot at a time.

2. Nutritional Sourcing: Providing Energy for the Body Temple

The basis of physical vitality is nutrition. Diets should be viewed as chances to nurture your body rather than as limitations. Accept a rainbow of vibrant fruits, veggies, nutritious grains, and lean meats. Staying hydrated is also important, so drink plenty of water.

Consider your body as a temple, and allow food to be a source of life, energy, and nourishment for your body.

3. Reflective Moments: The Efficaciousness of Rest

Embracing mindful moments in the midst of life's chaos is a powerful way to keep your body healthy. These peaceful times can be achieved through deep breathing, meditation, or just pausing to acknowledge the present. lower stress hormones, encourage deeper sleep, and improve general health. Building a foundation of mindfulness becomes essential to living a vital life.

4. Restorative Sleep: Rejuvenating the Body

The unsung hero of physical vigor is sleep. The nightly sleep is when the body repairs itself, regenerates, and consolidates memories. Make getting a good night's sleep a priority by setting up a regular sleep pattern, furnishing your bedroom with comfortable furnishings, and relaxing before bed. A body that has received enough sleep is alert and prepared to face the day's obstacles.

5. Social Networks: The Lifeblood of Society

Human connection is what keeps the body physically alive. Develop deep connections with others, look after your social network, and take part in activities that promote a feeling of community. The advantages of social ties on mental and physical health is significant; they serve as a stress reliever and promote a robust and full existence.

6. Playful Activities: Regaining Happiness

Remember to play in the search of physical vitality. Take part in joyful activities, such as sports, hobbies, or just spending time in nature. Playfulness enhances physical health and general well-being in addition to bringing interest to your routine. Rekindling the excitement of play maintains the body and spirit young.

The Vitality Blueprint: A Permanent Financial Commitment

Sustaining physical vitality is a lifetime adventure rather than a destination. It's a holistic strategy that includes taking care of one's body, mind, and spirit. Through combining exercise, meditation, mindful eating, and By incorporating excellent sleep, social relationships, and joyful pastimes into your daily routine, you establish a vitality blueprint that guarantees your body remains a robust and vibrant vessel for the experiences that await. Thus, go off on this path with enthusiasm, understanding that every action you take contributes to the longevity and vitality of your physical health.

COGNITIVE BENEFITS AND MENTAL AGILITY

The secret to cognitive advantages that go well beyond the norm lies in the human mind, which is like a vast and unexplored wilderness. Taking the journey to improve mental agility opens up a world where resilience, creativity, and problem-solving flourish. Let's explore the cognitive techniques and surprisingly beneficial effects that hold the key to revealing the complete potential of our complex mental landscape.

1. Brain Gymnastics: The Mental Exercise

Brain gymnastics enhances cognitive capacities in the same way that exercise strengthens the body. Games, crosswords, and puzzles test mental flexibility, or neuroplasticity—the brain's capacity to rearrange and adapt. Frequent mental exercises ensure a robust and flexible mind by improving memory and problem-solving abilities as well as helping to build new brain connections.

2. Education Journeys: Widening Brain Boundaries

Adopting a continual learning mindset opens up new brain boundaries with every new piece of knowledge, creating a cognitive adventure. Learning is a brain-stirring activity that can involve learning a new language, taking up an instrument, or pursuing an interest. It not only improves memory but also cultivates flexibility, critical thinking, and a quick-witted attitude to overcoming the challenges of daily life.

3. Reflective Moments: The Soothing Salve for Mental Instability

Including mindful moments in the hectic pace of modern life acts as a calming salve for mental flexibility. In addition to lowering stress, techniques like mindfulness and meditation improve focus, attention, and cognitive flexibility. The capacity to remain in the present moment sharpens the mind's reaction to difficulties, generating a mental environment that is robust and flexible.

4. The Strategic Game of Social Chess: Interactions

In addition to being essential for emotional health, social relationships provide mental agility with a tactical playground. The brain is forced to assimilate information, comprehend viewpoints, and adjust to changing social cues when participating in meaningful conversations, managing social dynamics, and building connections. Playing social chess can enhance cognitive abilities by strengthening interpersonal intelligence and fostering empathy.

5. The Creative Odyssey: Fostering Originality

The compass that leads the mind on an exciting journey is creativity. Whether via creative endeavors, puzzles, or experimentation with new concepts, nourishing creativity promotes cognitive adaptability. It fosters creativity and guarantees mental flexibility in the face of constantly changing circumstances by pushing the mind to approach problems from a variety of perspectives. 6. Restorative Sleep: Enhancing Cognitive Ability

Amid the chaos of everyday existence, getting enough sleep turns out to be an essential weapon for preserving mental toughness. The brain renews cognitive capabilities, processes emotions, and consolidates memories as you sleep. Making a healthy sleep a priority is like giving the mind the replenishment it needs to function at its best and be mentally flexible all day.

The Odyssey of the Mind: A Lifetime Journey

Advantages related to cognition and mental flexibility are not final goals, but rather an ongoing journey through the vast territories of the mind. You set out on a path that promises a robust, flexible, and dynamic mental landscape by combining brain gymnastics, accepting lifelong learning, engaging in mindfulness practices, managing social relationships, encouraging creativity, and placing a high priority on getting enough sleep. The journey takes place in the decisions you make on a daily basis, unleashing the power of your intellect and setting out on a journey of cognition that goes beyond the realm of the commonplace.

LONGEVITY SECRETS FROM AROUND THE WORLD

Numerous communities worldwide recognized for their exceptional longevity have ingrained a wealth of wisdom into their lifestyles, which is why the pursuit of a longer and better life is a topic of great interest to people everywhere. Discover the fascinating longevity secrets that cut across continents and cultures, from the tranquil islands of Okinawa to the sun-kissed highlands of Ikaria.

1. Okinawa, Japan: Hara Hachi Bu's Power

The idea of "Hara Hachi Bu" is central to the serene embrace of Okinawa, a small island in Japan. It means to eat till 80% satisfied, which is a deeply rooted custom in Okinawan culture. The Okinawans eat a diet high in vegetables, tofu, and sweet potatoes and practice mindful eating, which helps them consume fewer calories and, astonishingly, have some of the longest lifespans. lifetimes on our planet.

2. Greece's Ikaria: The Mediterranean Cure

Mediterranean cuisine is king in sun-kissed Ikaria, an island paradise in the Aegean Sea. Rich in fresh vegetables, legumes, olive oil, and a hint of red wine, this diet is not only a source of delicious food but also an essential component of long life. The Ikarians place a high value on relaxed living, afternoon naps, and social interactions—a trifecta that promotes both physical and emotional health.

3. The Pura Vida Lifestyle on Costa Rica's Nicoya Peninsula

The Pura Vida way of life flourishes on the Nicoya Peninsula's verdant surroundings. This Costa Rican philosophy, which translates as "pure life," places a great emphasis on social cohesion, simplicity, and a connection to the natural world. The Nicoyans eat a diet high in beans and exercise on a regular basis. and grain, and embrace life with a purpose—a blend that creates the fabric of their prolonged lives.

4. Take a sip from the Fountain of Youth in Sardinia, Italy

Longevity is no mystery on the picture-perfect island of Sardinia, where the aroma of Mediterranean herbs fills the air. Sardinians eat a diet rich in whole grains, veggies, and cheese made from goat's milk. Their strong work ethic, emphasis on family, and tight-knit communities all contribute to a way of life that eludes aging.

5. Loma Linda, California: America's Blue Zone

The city of Loma Linda, which is located in a Blue Zone—a place where people live longer, healthier lives—stands out in the center of Southern California. The majority of the people are Seventh-day Adventists, who follow a a plant-based diet, place an emphasis on getting regular exercise, and enjoy a day off for introspection and relaxation. Their lifestyle selections demonstrate the powerful impact of a holistic approach to health and wellness.

6. Ogliastra, Sardinia: The Shepherds' Secrets of a Century Ago

A remarkable community of 100-year-old shepherds in the hilly region of Ogliastra, Sardinia, shares the keys to their longevity. These hardy people are a testament to the balance between a healthy diet, exercise, and a connection to the land. They live physically demanding lives caring to flocks and following a traditional diet of complete grains, dairy products, and locally grown food.

The World Wide Web of Life Expectancy

Though the specifics of longevity secrets differ between these varied places, a few themes come through: purposeful living, physical activity, strong social ties, and mindful nutrition. The worldwide fabric of Cultural customs, food preferences, and lifestyle decisions that support the possibility of living a longer, healthier life are all intertwined with longevity. The quest for longevity becomes a global adventure as we take inspiration from these many sources, embracing the cumulative knowledge of civilizations all around the world

CHAPTER FOUR

Age is just a number in the vast scheme of things, and adopting a youthful perspective is the key to releasing an eternal vitality. The spring of youth is not only in the physical realm but also in our perception, thought process, and approach to the world. Together, we will investigate how to develop an attitude that resists aging and creates an eternal spring inside.

1. Unleashed Curiosity: The Fountain of Youth

An unquenchable curiosity—an passion to explore, learn, and discover—lies at the core of a youthful attitude. Adopt a mindset of constant learning and actively seek out new experiences, pastimes, and information. In addition to maintaining mental agility, curiosity enriches each moment with the magic of limitless possibilities. establishing a constant springtime inside the spirit.

2. Optimism as Protection: The Luminance of Happiness

Optimism is the sunlight that dries up the old mentality seeds. Maintain an optimistic attitude by viewing obstacles as chances for personal development and failures as stepping stones to achievement. Optimism is a brilliant light that not only brightens your way but also generates a magnetic energy that draws happiness and fortitude, cultivating an outlook that is beyond temporal constraints.

3. Playful Spirit: Joyful Dancing

A young mentality embraces a joyful attitude and dances with enthusiasm. Take part in things that make you smile, laugh, and feel like you're having fun. Enjoying goofy moments, dancing in the rain, or finding happiness in the little things in life, A sense of playfulness keeps the soul eternally young and the heart light.

4. Resilience as the Source: Regaining Composure with Grace

There will always be ups and downs in life, and resilience is the wellspring from which a positive, optimistic outlook springs. Accept difficulties with poise, recover from failures with fortitude, and see hardship as a chance for personal development. Resilient thinking turns challenges into learning opportunities and keeps the spirit steady and evergreen.

5. Wonder Connection: Taking Care of the Inner Child

Young people have an open mind and a connection to their inner child, which allows them to see the world with wonder and open eyes. Rekindle the wonder of everyday experiences, take in the beauty all around you, and approach life with the wonder of a child discovering the globe for the initial instance. Keeping the sense of amazement alive keeps the mind and heart open to the wonders of life.

6. Adventure Spirit: Venturing Into the Unknown

The joy of exploring the unknown and the thrill of adventure are what feed a young mind. Step outside of your comfort zone, take risks, and have a bold attitude toward life. An adventurous soul keeps the spirit alive by taking on new challenges and journeys on a whim, turning every day into a new chapter in the vast tale of life.

The Inner Fountain of Youth

Age is only an illusion in the mind; the key to eternal youth is in the decisions we make every day. Maintaining a childlike perspective is about accepting time with an eternally youthful attitude, not about resisting its passage. We can access the everlasting spring that exists inside us by bringing curiosity, optimism, playfulness, resilience, wonder, and a dash of adventure into our lives. This mindset transcends time and embraces the endless possibilities of a life well-lived.

THE POWER OF POSITIVE THINKING

In the complex dance of life, the amazing power of positive thinking is frequently highlighted. This power extends beyond simple optimism to encompass many aspects of our lives. Discover the fascinating mechanics of this mindset-changing approach and how positive thinking may show the way to success, resiliency, and general well-being.

1. The Mind as a Garden: Fostering Happiness

Consider the mind to be a garden full with seeds, with thoughts as the seeds. Good thoughts are like the sun, fostering the development of vivid, strong ideas. People may create an environment that not only blooms with optimism but also bears the fruits of creativity, resilience, and a resilient spirit by tending to a garden of positivity.

2. Optimism as a Strengthener of Resilience

Fundamental to In order to embrace optimism as a resilience enhancer, one must engage in optimistic thinking. Positive thinkers are more prone to see obstacles as transient and overcomeable when faced with problems. This constant optimism serves as a beacon of hope, enabling people to face hardships head-on and overcome setbacks with newfound fortitude.

3. Mental Alchemy: Creating Opportunities Out of Difficulties

By working like mental alchemy, positive thought turns obstacles into chances for development. Those who have an optimistic outlook see challenges as opportunities for growth rather than as impassable impediments. This kind of thinking opens doors to creativity, problem-solving abilities, and the ability to use setbacks as opportunities for growth on both a personal and professional level.

4. Harmonious Health: Positive Thoughts and Well-Being

The relationship between The physical and mental aspects of health are harmoniously symbiotic. Research indicates that preserving an optimistic perspective may help reduce stress, improve immunological response, and improve cardiovascular health. The mind-body connection emerges as a potent ally, proving that mental health isn't the only aspect of holistic health that depends on having a positive outlook.

5. Magnetic Energy: Drawing Chances and Achievements

Thinking positively creates a magnetic energy that draws possibilities and success. People that radiate positivity tend to surround themselves with a network of like-minded people, which fosters a collaborative, innovative, and achievement-oriented environment.

The conviction that success is not just possible but an unavoidable fact gives one the ability to draw favorable results.

6. Shaping Destinies Through Self-Fulfilling Prophecy

The notion of A self-fulfilling prophesy emphasizes how powerfully positive thinking may influence people's fates. People are more inclined to act in ways consistent with their views when they have self-confidence and an optimistic mindset. By taking the initiative, one can frequently initiate a series of events that culminate in the achievement of their dreams and ambitions.

Accepting the Light of Positivity

Positive thinking is a luminous thread that weaves achievement, resilience, and well-being into the larger picture of life. It takes more than simply keeping a constant smile on your face to cultivate an optimistic outlook that sees potential where others see constraints. Accepting the power of positive thought is a call to awaken one's potential and reveal avenues that lead to a higher a lively, contented, and purpose-driven existence

CULTIVATING CURIOSITY AND ADAPTABILITY

In the unpredictable terrain of life, developing curiosity and flexibility becomes a powerful combination that not only drives personal growth but also serves as a beacon of hope for those navigating the intricacies of today's world. Explore the intriguing relationship that exists between adaptability and curiosity, and how cultivating these traits may promote a growth-oriented attitude that lasts a lifetime.

1. Unleashing Curiosity: The Spark of Discovery

The spark that starts the flame of exploration and discovery is curiosity. It is the inbuilt need to comprehend, inquire about, and solve the puzzles that surround us. Developing curiosity is like unlocking new vistas for people, enabling them to go on an endless path of discovery, ingenuity, and intellectual growth.

2. Adaptability as a Changing Kind of Resilience In a world where things are changing all the time, adaptation turns into the dynamic resilience that

guarantees not only survival but also flourishing in the face of uncertainty. Those that are flexible alter their sails to the winds of change, much like nimble navigators. This trait gives people the confidence to take on hurdles head-on, change course when necessary, and see setbacks as chances for personal development rather than insurmountable roadblocks.

3. The Learning Loop: Adaptability Is Fueled by Curiosity

A symbiotic relationship—a learning loop where one feeds into the other—between curiosity and adaptation exists. People that are curious search out fresh information, viewpoints, and experiences. This flood of data serves as the starting point for adaptability as people incorporate these new realizations into their perspectives, honing their strategies, and expanding their ability to flourish in a variety of settings.

4. Accepting Uncertainty: Curiosity's Recreation Area

In the playground of the unknown, where people voluntarily step outside of their comfort zones, curiosity flourishes. It is the readiness to ponder "why" and "what if," cultivating an open-minded attitude toward the possibilities that come with uncertainty. Curiosity-driven people like the process of unraveling the unknown and transforming it into the familiar. They find delight in the voyage of discovery.

5. Innovation Emerges: The Blossom of Adaptability

Adaptability gives rise to creativity when people apply their experiences and knowledge to develop original solutions. Not only does an adaptable mindset welcome change, it actively looks for new chances for innovation. It turns obstacles into opportunities for innovative problem-solving, resulting in ground-breaking concepts and methods that advance success on both a personal and professional level.

6. Lifelong Learning: Inquisitiveness and Flexibility as Partners

Adaptability and curiosity work together to create the conditions for lifelong learning. People who are always learning, who look for new challenges, and who adjust to changing conditions are always improving themselves. This process of development serves as evidence of the transformational potential of an open-minded, flexible attitude.

The Lifelong Learning Synergy

The story of lifelong learning that arises from the cultivation of curiosity and adaptation is the story of personal and professional progress. It's an adventure into the uncharted, a dance with transformation, and a dedication to continuous improvement. People who cultivate these attributes not only improve their own lives but also foster a culture of creativity, resiliency, and ongoing progress—a synergy that advances us all. moving forward in the dynamic fabric of our shared experience.

OVERCOMING AGE-RELATED MENTAL BARRIERS

Age should not be a barrier in the mosaic of life, but rather a mark of knowledge and experience. However, society frequently places mental obstacles on aging, leading to self-imposed constraints that impede advancement in both the personal and professional spheres. Let's set out on a quest to eliminate these age-related mental obstacles by investigating methods for escaping social norms and realizing the limitless potential of a dynamic, age-defying mind.

1. Redefining Achievement: The Constantly Expanding Range

The expectation of success by a particular age in society is a common mental barrier related to age. Consider success as a lifelong adventure with an ever-expanding horizon rather than following preset deadlines. Accept the notion that accomplishments, development, and fulfillment can happen at any time of life, dispelling the myth that specific benchmarks must be reached. ought to be accomplished by a specific age.

2. Lifelong Learning: An Indestructible Interest

The myth that learning stops as one gets older leads to mental limitations. Adopt a mindset that values lifelong learning and believes that intellectual curiosity is ageless. Breaking down mental barriers and promoting a constantly changing mind, lifelong learning becomes the antidote to stagnation, whether it is by learning new skills, investigating varied subjects, or venturing into unfamiliar territory.

3. Adaptation Flexibility: Accepting Change

Age-related mental obstacles frequently show up as reluctance to adapt. Develop flexibility as a fundamental quality, understanding that it is essential to surmount obstacles, seize fresh chances, and prosper in ever-changing surroundings. Being able to change course and adapt becomes an effective strategy for breaking down mental obstacles and embracing life with fortitude and receptivity.

4. Adopting Technology: Building a Generational Bridge

For individuals who were not raised with technology at their disposal, the digital age might be frightening. However, age-related mental limitations can be overcome by seeing technology as a bridge rather than a barrier. Seize the chances that technology presents for interaction, education, and creativity. People can stay in touch with younger generations in this way, which promotes cooperation and understanding between them.

5. Mind-Body Balance: Properly NurturingAge-related stereotypes concerning mental and physical deterioration are common. The mental obstacles

related to aging are broken, nevertheless, when holistic well-being is prioritized through activities like regular exercise, mindfulness, and a healthy lifestyle. The integration of physical and mental well-being establishes a balanced basis for a robust and dynamic intellect.

6. Following Your Passions: Fanning the Inner Flames

Anger should never be put out of its fire by age. Developing interests, pastimes, and creative projects becomes a potent way to overcome mental obstacles. Unleashing creativity and passion creates a sense of purpose, demonstrating that the fire within can burn brightly at any age, whether it is through writing, painting, or taking up new activities.

The Emancipation of an Eternal Mind

It is a liberating experience to overcome age-related mental obstacles and realize that, like great wine, the mind can get better with age. It entails putting social norms to the test, accepting change, encouraging lifelong learning, and promoting holistic wellbeing. People who break free from these mental restrictions discover the limitless possibilities of an immortal mind—a mind that survives, changes, and stays bright in the face of constantly shifting circumstances.

CHAPTER FIVE

REVOLUTIONIZING NUTRITION FOR OPTIMAL AGING

The function of nutrition becomes a revolutionary force in the quest for healthy aging—a dynamic catalyst that can completely change our understanding of the aging process. Together, we will investigate cutting-edge tactics, dietary changes, and nutritional discoveries that transform how we fuel our bodies and guarantee not only long life but also a dynamic and healthy transition into old age.

1. The Nutrient Symphony: A Consistent Equilibrium

Understanding the nutrient symphony that our bodies yearn for is the first step toward revolutionizing nutrition for optimal aging. It entails adopting a nutritious, well-balanced diet high in vitamins, minerals, antioxidants, and other vital elements. The balance of nutrients promotes general resilience and well-being by acting as a barrier against age-related illnesses.

2. Functional Foods: The Cure for Extended Life Duration the era of functional foods, an innovative idea that goes beyond the need of basic sustenance. Including foods that have particular health benefits becomes essential to good aging. With their

ability to reduce inflammation and improve cognitive function, functional foods provide a tailored approach to nutrition that caters to the special requirements of aging bodies and brains.

3. Mindful Eating: An Innovative Technique

Improving nutrition involves not just what we eat but also how we eat. Introducing mindful eating, a novel strategy that places an emphasis on enjoying every bite, being aware of hunger indicators, and developing a stronger bond with the act of feeding oneself. Meals become joyful experiences because to this mindful revolution, which also improves digestion, vitamin absorption, and general satisfaction.

4. Protein Abundance: Essential Components for Energy

The body's need for protein increases with age. Transform your diet by realizing how important protein is for maintaining bone health, building muscle mass, and sustaining general health. Getting enough protein from both plant-based and lean meat sources is crucial for achieving ideal aging.

5. Microbiome Magic: The Revolution in Gut Health

A large community of bacteria found in our digestive tract, the gut microbiome is emerging as a revolutionary frontier in healthy aging. Prebiotics, probiotics, and fiber-rich diets become a weapon for supporting immune system performance, digestive health, and even mental clarity. A comprehensive strategy for ageing gracefully from the inside out is being pioneered by the gut health movement.

6. Hydration Renaissance: Fountain of Youth Hydration is the unsung hero of the nutrition revolution, taking center stage. For aging to be optimal, a resurgence of interest in hydration, with a focus on how crucial a sufficient water intake is for cellular health, skin health, and general vitality. A simple glass of water could be the key to eternal life, supporting the innovative goal of gracefully aging.

The Nutrition Revolution: A New Definition of Aging

Modernizing nutrition for the best possible aging process is a dynamic process of exploration and adaptation rather than a one-size-fits-all solution. It entails adopting cutting-edge nutritional techniques, accepting the most recent scientific discoveries, and cultivating an attitude that sees food as fuel for a full life. We are starting a nutritional revolution as we rethink how we feed our bodies. This revolution will go beyond the conventional notions of aging and guarantee that the golden years are not only endured but also cherished as a period of vigor, resilience, and continuous expansion.

ANTI-AGING FOODS AND NUTRIENTS

The importance of anti-aging foods and minerals takes center stage in the quest for ageless well-being as the desire for longevity and vigor gets traction. Discover the superfoods and vital nutrients that not only fuel the body but also contain the secrets to opening the fountain of youth as we go into the realm of nutritional alchemy.

1. Omega-3 Fatty Acids: Your Best Friend in the Brain

Omega-3 fatty acids, which are rich in walnuts, flaxseeds, and fatty fish like salmon, are powerful friends in the battle against aging. These necessary fats promote healthy brain function, lower inflammatory levels, and promote smooth, glowing skin. You're strengthening your cognitive abilities in addition to providing nourishment for your body when you include foods high in omega-3 fatty acids in your diet.

2. Vibrant Berries Packed with Antioxidants: Nature's Anti-Aging Supplement

Berries, with their vivid colors, are a gift from nature to everyone looking for nutrition that defies aging. Berries, which are rich in antioxidants called anthocyanins, help to maintain skin suppleness, lower inflammation, and fight oxidative stress. Strawberries, raspberries, and blueberries turn into a powerful potion that supports cellular longevity and health in addition to being a delectable snack.

3. Leafy Greens: The Superfoods of Nutrients

In the realm of anti-aging, dark, leafy greens such as Swiss chard, kale, and spinach are like superheroes. Packed with vitamins, minerals, and antioxidants, these greens help maintain strong bones, strengthen the immune system, and help keep skin looking young. Greens' natural detoxifying agent, chlorophyll, aids in the body's removal of pollutants and preservation of healthy cell function.

4. Turmeric: The Longevity Spice Due to its active ingredient curcumin, emerges as the golden spice of longevity. Renowned for its anti-inflammatory and antioxidant properties, turmeric offers a multitude of health benefits. From joint health to cognitive function, incorporating turmeric into your diet or enjoying golden milk becomes a flavorful strategy for combating the wear and tear of aging.

5. Nuts and Seeds: Tiny Packages of Age-Defying Goodness

Nuts and seeds, whether almonds, sunflower seeds, or chia seeds, are nutritional powerhouses brimming with anti-aging goodness. Packed with omega-3 fatty acids, vitamins, and minerals, these tiny packages contribute to heart health, skin elasticity, and overall well-being. Snacking on a handful of nuts or adding seeds to your meals becomes a delightful ritual with long-lasting benefits.

6. Protein-Rich Quinoa: A Grain for Radiant Aging

Quinoa, hailed as a full protein, is unique in that it encourages glowing aging. Quinoa's remarkable amino acid composition promotes tissue regeneration, muscle health, and long-term energy. Quinoa becomes a mainstay in the anti-aging pantry due to its versatility and high vitamin content, which promotes cellular and physical vitality.

7. Green Tea: Drinking Eternity

Green tea is the beverage of choice for those who wish to live longer and look younger because of its high antioxidant content. Green tea, which is high in polyphenols, improves metabolism, strengthens the heart, and has anti-aging properties. Drinking green tea makes drinking it a pleasurable routine that gives you the energy of youth all day long.

Accepting Anti-Aging Eating as a Lifestyle Option

The secret to the harmony of anti-aging foods and nutrients is not just the components alone, but also the combination they produce in a well-rounded, balanced diet. Accepting these foods that defy aging becomes more than just a decision about what to eat; it becomes a way of life that supports your body and your pursuit of resilience, vigor, and an enduring sense of well-being. Unlock these nutritional gems' potential to become a more young, radiant version of yourself.

IMPORTANCE OF HYDRATION AND SKIN HEALTH

Hydration emerges as an underappreciated hero in the complex dance of self-care. Sufficient hydration is not just essential for life support; it is also the key to healthy, glowing skin. Let's explore the significance of hydration and how it serves as the basis for a comprehensive strategy for maintaining skin health, opening the door to a radiant complexion and ageless beauty.

1. Water is the Fountain of Youth and the Skin's Lifeline

Think of water as the paintbrush that creates a vibrant picture on your skin. The key to preserving the skin's overall resilience, suppleness, and elasticity is being hydrated. Maintaining proper hydration of the skin results in a canvas that resists the effects of aging and promotes a young glow that lasts a lifetime.

2. An Organic Glow: Internal Hydration

Although skincare products are important, inside hydration is where the real magic happens. Getting enough water into your diet on a regular basis is like giving your skin a revitalizing drink. Within-based hydration nourishes skin cells, eliminates toxins, and adds to a naturally beautiful glow that is unmatched by topical creams.

3. Hydration's Impact on Wrinkle Reduction: Plump and Supple

Hydration has the superpower of minimising the look of fine lines and wrinkles. Skin that is well-hydrated is supple and plump, which reduces the appearance of wrinkles caused by aging. It's as though you're giving your skin a natural filler, thanks to the small but significant action of drinking enough water.

4. Barrier Function: Protecting the Skin from Environmental Factors and Moisture serves to reinforce the skin's barrier function by acting as a shield of protection. A moisturized skin barrier is more resilient to UV radiation, contaminants, and environmental stressors. It's like arming your skin with strong armor, making sure it stays a rock-solid protector against the everyday barrage of outside aggressors.

5. Dispelling Boredom: The Illuminating Effect of Hydration

Skin that is dehydrated frequently has a lifeless, bland complexion. On the other hand, skin that is adequately hydrated has a glowing quality. It improves light reflection, which gives your skin a radiant, healthy glow that transcends simple attractiveness.

6. Treating Common Skin Conditions: Eczema, Acne, and More

Hydration is a salve for many skin conditions. It contributes to controlling oil production by assisting in the prevention of outbreaks of acne. Sustaining proper hydration becomes a calming cure for those suffering from skin diseases such as rosacea, psoriasis, or eczema, as it eases irritation and promotes overall skin health.

7. Wholesome Hydration: Exceeding Water Consumption

Although drinking enough water is important, comprehensive hydration goes beyond this. An all-encompassing strategy includes using hydrating skincare products, eating foods high in water, and limiting your intake of alcohol and caffeine. The combination of external and internal moisture becomes the magic formula for a long-lasting skin care routine.

Taking Care of Inner Beauty

Hydration appears as a narrative thread woven within the everlasting beauty of the larger story of self-care. Water consumption is only one aspect of a lifestyle decision that supports your internal skin. You may start your road toward a complexion that exudes resilience, energy, and the ageless beauty that comes from a well-hydrated, luminous canvas by realizing the crucial connection between hydration and skin health. Drink in this hydration elixir and see how your skin becomes a work of lasting beauty.

THE ROLE OF EXERCISE IN AGING BACKWARD

In the vast story of life, when time seems to be moving on with unrelenting determination, there is a potent remedy—a recipe that breaks with convention—that can be found. Exercise is that magic bullet, and it can truly improve one's aging process. Together, we can uncover the deep effects of physical activity and rewrite the tale of aging to tell one of vitality, resiliency, and enduring well-being. Let's set out on this journey.

1. Muscle Magic: Creating a Younger Body

The aging process is characterized by a loss of muscle mass as the years pass. But consistent exercise, particularly strength training, works like a magic wand to shape and preserve muscle mass. Not only is it aesthetically pleasing, but it's also an important tactic for preserving strength, balance, and the capacity for agile movement—qualities necessary for a young, active life.

2. Second, Bone Density Ballet: Preventing Osteoporosis

Over time, there is a gradual loss of bone density that can result in diseases such as osteoporosis. Exercise— especially resistance training and weightlifting—becomes the bone-fortifying choreography. It's a ballet that prevents breaks, making sure the skeleton is strong and resilient while resembling youth's grace.

3. Cardiovascular Symphony: The Youth's Heartbeat

Cardiovascular exercise helps the heart, the rhythmic maestro of our body, age gracefully. Exercises that raise the heart rate, like swimming, jogging, or brisk walking, produce a cardiovascular symphony. It keeps the heart beating by improving circulation, lowering the risk of heart disease, and fostering endurance. to the tune of youth.

4. Brain Gym: Developing Cognitive Acuity

Exercise is a mental gymnastics routine as well as a physical activity. Regular physical activity has been shown in studies to improve memory, increase mental clarity overall, and raise cognitive performance. It's a spring of youth for our minds, reminding us that physical activity nourishes our brains, the fundamental source of our brilliance.

5. Flexibility Ballet: Grasping Elegant Motions

One frequently has a sense of stiffness and decreased flexibility as they age. Now for the flexibility ballet, a routine that combines yoga, stretching, and conscious motions. These exercises not only improve flexibility but also support healthy joints, allowing the body to move gracefully and fluidly, resembling its youthful suppleness.

6. Mood Elevation Symphony: A Spiritual Serenade

Exercise is like a mood-altering symphony, with the lovely notes of endorphins soothing the soul. It relieves tension, eases anxiety, and is a natural antidepressant. Exercise's psychological advantages support a positive outlook, emotional fortitude, and a sense of wellbeing that lasts beyond the number of years.

7. Tango Telomere: Dissecting the Molecular Clock

Telomeres, the protective caps on the ends of chromosomes, are markers of the molecular clock located deep within our cells. Exercise seems to help maintain telomere length, which slows down the aging process of cells. At the molecular level, exercise is like a tango, where the dance unwraps the clock and reminds us that age is more than just a number.

The Reverse Journey: Graceful Aging and Vitality

In the pursuit of aging backward, exercise emerges not as a grueling task but as a transformative journey—one that rewires the narrative of aging and reveals the profound connection between movement and vitality. It's a journey that transcends traditional notions of getting older, inviting us to embrace a life marked by strength, resilience, and the timeless spirit of youth. So, lace up those sneakers, embark on the journey, and let the symphony of exercise guide you in rewriting the script of aging.

CHAPTER SIX

SOCIAL CONNECTIONS AND EMOTIONAL WELL-BEING

The Art of Social Connection: A Route to Mental Health and Happiness

The complex web of social connection is woven across the vast tapestry of human existence and our daily existence. It is a thread that unites us, weaves across our lives, and tints the canvas of our mental health. The significance of authentic human connection is immeasurable in a society where chaos frequently reigns.

Empathy, comprehension, and the sharing of common experiences are at the core of social connection. It's the understated language of a consoling touch, the sincere warmth of a smile, and the resonance of real discussion. The soul is nourished by these moments of connection, which create an acceptance and belonging that is beyond words. by themselves.

Studies have demonstrated the significant influence that social connections have on mental health. Research continuously shows that those with strong social support systems are better able to deal with life's obstacles and report reduced levels of stress, anxiety, and sadness.

Furthermore, the impact of connection goes beyond emotional fortitude to include physical and cognitive well-being as well as general quality of life.

The social connection landscape has changed in the current digital era, presenting both novel obstacles and hitherto unseen opportunities. Through social media, we can communicate with each other and others on different countries, celebrate our successes, and ask for help when we need it. However, despite the appeal of virtual connection, there is a painful paradox: the more linked we are to the internet, the more likely it is that we will lose sight of the depth of and genuineness that come with in-person communication.

To foster real connections in the midst of modernity's cacophony, one must be purposeful and present. It's about securing times of mutual vulnerability, developing empathy, and appreciating the beauty in human frailty. The seeds of real connection are sown when we listen intently, speak from the heart, and show kindness without expecting anything in return.

In addition to improving our personal lives, social connection enriches the fabric of the human experience as a whole. Communities based on inclusivity and empathy become havens of support where people are given the tools they need to prosper. Compassion, resiliency, and communal well-being are the seeds that find rich soil in these dynamic ecosystems of connection and grow. expand.

Let's value social connection as a fundamental component of emotional health as we negotiate the intricacies of a globalized society. Let's reach out, cross gaps, and create understanding bridges that cut beyond generations, cultures, and ideologies. Because our connections—with ourselves, with others, and with the outside world—are what weave the threads of human existence together and show us the way to great fulfillment, healing, and wholeness.

BUILDING MEANINGFUL RELATIONSHIPS

There is an artistry in the complex dance of human interaction—a delicate interlacing of threads that creates the fabric of meaningful connections. These relationships, which are cultivated via mutual respect, understanding, and shared experiences, strengthen our bonds and give our life meaning and purpose. A path of self-discovery, openness, and genuine connection is revealed when one examines the fundamentals of creating lasting connections.

Acknowledging Authenticity: The foundation of any lasting connection is the bravery to be genuine to who we are, flaws and all, without fear of criticism or rejection. Sincerity and mutual respect are the foundations of intimacy and trust, and authenticity enables us to establish connections based on these qualities.

Fostering Compassion and Understanding: Compassion acts as a link between us and the lived experiences of other people, encouraging empathy, and strengthening emotional ties. Relationships can grow when we foster an atmosphere of empathy by actively listening, attempting to understand, and validating one another's viewpoints.

Handling Conflict with Grace: While conflict is an inherent part of any relationship, it also offers a chance for development and a better knowledge of one another. Disagreements can become opportunities to deepen our relationships if we approach them with humility, understanding, and a readiness to have frank conversations.

Promoting Mutual Support and Encouragement: Mutual support, encouragement, and affirmation are mutually exchanged in meaningful relationships, which are defined by a spirit of reciprocity. Through rejoicing in each other's accomplishments, lending a sympathetic ear when necessary, and remaining resilient throughout difficult times, we foster a feeling of community and unity that nourishes the spirit.

Taking Care of Shared Experiences and Memories: Our relationships are defined by the moments that weave together our shared experiences, which serve as a foundation for our memories. Whether via misadventures, giggles, or quiet times for introspection, these common experiences serve as the cornerstone around which enduring relationships are constructed.

Respecting Boundaries and Individuality: Building wholesome, long-lasting relationships requires a respect for boundaries and individual liberty. People feel appreciated, respected, and free to express themselves genuinely when we respect each other's needs, preferences, and personal space.

Cultivating Appreciation and Gratitude: Meaningful relationships are built on gratitude, which serves as a reminder to treasure the beauty of connection and show appreciation for the contributions people make to our lives. lives. We strengthen our ties to one another and foster a culture of appreciation for one another when we recognize the efforts of people we care about and show our sincere gratitude.

The art of creating lasting connections rests at the crossroads of genuine connection, empathy, and vulnerability in the tapestry of human experience. Let's embrace the richness of human connection as we set out on this voyage of research and discovery, cultivating relationships that profoundly and meaningfully inspire, uplift, and enrich our lives.

EMOTIONAL RESILIENCE AND COPING STRATEGIES

Getting Through Life's Storms: The Value of Coping Mechanisms and Emotional Resilience

The intricacy of life throws us a wide range of obstacles; some are expected, some are not. Emotional resilience shows up as our reliable ally in the midst of hardship, enabling us to navigate choppy waters and tackle life's challenges head-on with courage and grace. A path to resilience, strength, and personal development can be found by comprehending the fundamentals of emotional resilience and adopting useful coping mechanisms.

Accepting Adversity as a Growth-Catalyst: Even in its most intimidating forms, adversity harbors the potential for growth and adaptability. We equip ourselves to face life's curveballs with bravery and resiliency when we reframe obstacles as chances for development and learning.

Developing Self-Awareness and Mindfulness: Fundamental to The foundation of emotional resilience is a strong sense of self-awareness, or the capacity to accept and acknowledge our feelings without opposition or condemnation. We develop an inner calm and sense of presence through mindfulness exercises like deep breathing, body awareness, and meditation that work as a guiding light during trying moments.

Creating a Network of Relationships That may Support You: Human connection is essential to emotional resilience because it may provide comfort, affirmation, and assistance when needed. We establish a safety net of support that increases our resilience and gives us a sense of belonging by cultivating connections based on trust, empathy, and respect for one another.

Using Adaptive Coping methods: Using adaptive coping methods helps us face challenges head-on and handle them gracefully and resiliently, preventing us from giving up or losing hope. Solving problems, looking for social support, using creative outlets, and discovering meaning and purpose in the face of hardship are a few examples of these tactics.

Developing Optimism and Gratitude: These two emotions provide our life a sense of possibility, hope, and resilience, making them effective counterbalances to pessimism. Our viewpoint changes from one of scarcity to one of abundance when we learn to see the bright spots in life and develop a thankfulness attitude for all the things we have.

Realistic Goal-Setting and Expectations: By establishing realistic goals and expectations, we can avoid burnout or overwhelm and instead face life's obstacles with clarity and purpose. By dissecting more ambitious objectives into more manageable chunks and acknowledging tiny victories along the way, we foster a feeling of autonomy and success that supports our journey toward resiliency.

Acceptance and Self-Compassion: Self-compassion becomes a light in our darkest moments, providing us with comfort, understanding, and acceptance. We may develop an inner strength and resilience that endures hardship by being kind to ourselves, accepting our flaws and vulnerabilities with grace, and treating ourselves with care.

Emotional resilience appears as a beacon of hope in the human experience, a reflection of the heart's unwavering spirit. As we make our way through the maze of life, let's embrace the strength of emotional resilience and develop useful coping mechanisms that will enable us to meet obstacles head-on with bravery, grace, and unshakeable resilience.

LAUGHTER, JOY, AND THE FOUNTAIN OF YOUTH

Laughter and joy are two of the brightest threads in the vast fabric of human existence. These two friends, who are joyfully dancing down our life's hallways, are the key to an eternal potion known as the Fountain of Youth. We are going to go on a voyage of exploration, amazement, and unbounded vigor as we learn about the enormous effects that joy and laughing have on our physical, mental, and spiritual health.

The Healing Power of Humor: Laughter is a tonic for the body and a balm for the spirit because of its contagious charm and unplanned joy. Hearts become lighter, tensions release, and stress disappears in its embrace. Research has indicated that laughing strengthens the immune system and causes the release of endorphins, which are nature's own mood enhancers. This leaves us feeling refreshed and revived.

Developing Joy as a Mode of Being: Joy speaks to us of the innate beauty and wonder of life, like a soft summer wind. It is a way of being, not just a feeling, that is developed via mindfulness, gratitude, and a profound appreciation for the here and now. We discover ourselves completely awake and attuned to the surrounding symphony of reality when we are in the embrace of joy.

Establishing Connections Through Mutual Laughter: Laughter's ability to unite people crosses barriers and creates bridges across countries, languages, and generations. Strangers become friends and differences seem insignificant when they laugh together. We uncover the humanity that unites us via laughter, like a tapestry stitched with threads. of happiness and friendship.

Embracing a youngster's Wonder and Playfulness: A youngster sees the world as an endless playground, a blank canvas waiting to be filled with fantasies and experiences. We rediscover the wonder of discovery, the magic of creativity, and the joy of small pleasures when we embrace our inner kid. Playfulness allows us to break free from the limitations of maturity and allows spontaneity and creativity to enter our lives.

Embracing Joy and Laughter in Daily Life: The pursuit of joy and laughter frequently takes a backseat to commitments and responsibilities in the rush of daily life. However, among the mayhem, there is a call to look for humorous moments, find humor in the ordinary, and accept human ridiculousness. expertise. Let us enjoy the delicacy of joy and laughter in all of its manifestations, whether via a sincere belly laugh, a joke between friends, or an impromptu dance.

Let us follow the invitation to laugh and rejoice as we navigate the kaleidoscope of life—the never-ending spring from which youth springs. We find the essence of life, the key to a life well lived, and the limitless enchantment of the human spirit in their embrace. We discover the real key to perpetual youth in the dance of laughter and joy, so let's laugh unreservedly, love completely, and welcome every moment with open arms.

CHAPTER SEVEN

FINANCIAL AND LIFESTYLE FREEDOM

In the midst of modern existence, the pursuit of financial and lifestyle freedom serves as a light of hope—a promise of emancipation from the confines of convention and the shackles of scarcity. As we engage on this voyage of research and empowerment, we will discover the keys to living a life of plenty, meaning, and fulfillment.

Financial Empowerment: Beyond the Balance Sheet. Financial freedom is more than just numbers on a balance sheet; it is a condition of empowerment, a declaration of control over one's economic future. It is the ability to follow passions, goals, and live life on one's own terms, free of financial concerns or constraints.

Redefining Success: Beyond Material Wealth. In order to achieve financial freedom, we must reframe our definitions of success—recognizing that true richness goes well beyond material prosperity. It can be found in the breadth of experiences, the depth of relationships, and the pursuit of passions that energize the spirit. It is the freedom to live truthfully, pursue purpose-driven goals, and develop a meaningful and significant existence.

Embracing Minimalism and Intentional Living: At the heart of lifestyle freedom is the idea of minimalism, which emphasizes simplicity, intentionality, and mindful consumerism. By decluttering our lives, both materially and emotionally, we make room for what is actually important, shedding excess and embracing the essence of what brings us joy, contentment, and freedom.

Creating Multiple Streams of revenue: Diversifying our revenue streams allows us to break free from the constraints of traditional employment, resulting in financial prosperity and entrepreneurial independence. Whether through passive income investments, freelance projects, or internet company initiatives, the goal of financial freedom transforms into a voyage of creativity, invention, and boundless opportunity.

Cultivating Financial Literacy and clever: Financial freedom is a journey, not a destination. It is paved with financial literacy, clever decision-making, and disciplined resource stewardship. By investing in financial knowledge, developing smart money management skills, and adopting an abundance mindset, we establish the groundwork for a prosperous and secure future.

Prioritizing Health and Well-Being: True lifestyle freedom entails not only financial prosperity but also holistic well-being—nurturing the body, mind, and spirit in accordance with natural cycles and intuition. By putting health, self-care, and personal growth first, we promote a life of vitality, resilience, and deep fulfillment.

Fostering Connection and Contribution: In the search of freedom, we are urged to acknowledge our interconnectedness—to create deep, meaningful relationships while also contributing to the well-being of others and the globe. The genuine core of abundance is found in the spirit of service, generosity, and empathy—the freedom to give, receive, and make a meaningful difference in people's lives.

As we explore the great expanse of possibilities that awaits us, let us view the pursuit of financial and lifestyle independence as a sacred journey—one of self-discovery, empowerment, and deep transformation. Pursuing our innermost desires and highest principles opens the way to a life of limitless opportunity, infinite potential, and unmatched freedom.

REDEFINING RETIREMENT

Retirement, historically associated with peace and relaxation, is undergoing a significant transition in today's dynamic world. Retirement is no longer constrained to a typical narrative of leisurely hobbies and quiet introspection; it is becoming a vibrant chapter of exploration, reinvention, and meaningful living. As we redefine retirement, we start on a voyage of discovery— one that embraces the richness of experience, the pursuit of passions, and the human spirit's limitless potential.

Embracing lifetime Learning: In the new retirement landscape, learning becomes a lifetime pursuit—a chance to broaden horizons, gain new skills, and engage in intellectual inquiry. Retirement allows you to pursue areas of curiosity and interest, whether through formal education, online courses, or hands-on experiences, developing the mind and nurturing the soul.

Pursuing Passion Projects: Retirement marks the beginning of a new era—a time to rekindle passions, pursue long-held aspirations, and immerse oneself in creative projects. Retirement serves as a blank canvas for self-expression and fulfillment, enjoying the joy of creation and the thrill of discovery.

Purposeful Work: For many people, retirement is not the end of work, but rather the beginning of a new chapter of meaningful engagement. Retirement provides possibilities to have a good influence, contribute to causes of personal significance, and leave a legacy of service and compassion, whether through part-time employment, volunteer activities, or community involvement.

Cultivating Health and Well-Being: Retirement gives you the gift of time—the opportunity to prioritize your health, wellbeing, and self-care. Retirement allows you to nurture your body, mind, and spirit, building a sense of vitality, resilience, and inner peace via regular exercise and thoughtful activities like yoga and meditation.

Building and Maintaining Relationships: Retirement allows us to cultivate stronger connections with loved ones, friends, and communities. It is a time to appreciate the simple pleasures of company, to make enduring memories, and to treasure the relationships that enrich our lives. Retirement, whether through travel, shared experiences, or sincere talks, becomes a time to celebrate connection and belonging.

Embracing Financial Planning and Security: As we redefine retirement, financial planning becomes more important—a road map to security, stability, and peace of mind. From sensible investments to budgeting tactics and retirement savings, financial planning enables us to face life's uncertainties with confidence and resilience, ensuring that our retirement years are filled with richness and freedom.

Celebrating Diversity and inclusiveness: As retirement approaches, diversity and inclusiveness emerge as guiding principles—a celebration of the complexity of the human experience and the worth of each individual. Retirement becomes an opportunity to embrace diversity, cultivate inclusivity, and build communities in which everyone is welcomed, respected, and valued for their unique contributions.

Redefining retirement is more than a mental shift; it demonstrates the human spirit's persistence and adaptability. It is a proclamation of possibility—a promise to live life to the fullest, to embrace new experiences, and to appreciate the beauty of each moment. As we embark on this path of rediscovery and regeneration, let us embrace retirement's limitless possibilities and relish the richness of experience that awaits us on this magnificent voyage called life.

PURSUING PASSION PROJECTS AT ANY AGE

Passion projects are a powerful tool for personal growth, exploration, and self-discovery. They allow us to tap into our innate creativity, nurture lifelong learning, and embrace the spirit of exploration. These projects offer a platform for experimentation, innovation, and pushing the boundaries of what is possible. They also teach resilience and perseverance, enabling us to grow and evolve. Passion projects also provide a sense of purpose and meaning, connecting us with our deepest values and aspirations. They also foster connections and community, enriching our lives and nourishing our souls. The journey of passion projects is celebrated, not just the destination, as it celebrates the beauty of creativity, the joy of discovery, and the transformative power of following our hearts. As we embark on this journey, let us embrace the beauty of the creative process, the joy of exploration, and the fulfillment that comes from following our hearts.

THE ART OF BALANCING WORK AND LEISURE

In the journey of life, finding the right mix between work and leisure sets the tone for our daily rhythm. Just like skilled conductors, we guide ourselves through the ups and downs, looking for harmony amidst our responsibilities and times of relaxation. Balancing work and leisure isn't just about managing time; it's about embracing a profound dance—one that celebrates our experiences, successes, and inner well-being.

Engaging with Work as Meaningful Contribution: Work goes beyond a simple task—it shows our sense of purpose, passion, and desire to contribute. Whether in our careers, academic pursuits, or creative endeavors, work helps us to deeply engage with the world, making meaningful impacts and utilizing our talents for the better good.

Practicing Mindful Presence in Work and Play: Mindfulness gives a sense of awareness to both our work and leisure activities. It encourages us to fully immerse ourselves in each moment, whether we're in a meeting or having leisure time outdoors. Mindfulness helps us appreciate the beauty of the moment and stay connected to the world around us.

Setting Healthy Boundaries and Priorities: Achieving balance requires setting clear boundaries and priorities. It's about recognizing the value of productivity as well as relaxation and making room for both in our lives. By setting limits around work commitments and prioritizing activities that nourish our bodies, minds, and souls, we find equilibrium in our daily routines.

Encouraging Creativity and Exploration: Leisure provides an avenue for creativity and discovery—a place where we can freely express ourselves and explore new interests. Whether through art, outdoor adventures, or intellectual hobbies, leisure time allows us to expand our horizons, follow our passions, and revel in the joy of discovery.

Nurturing Relationships and Connection: Both work and leisure are enriched by the ties we cultivate—with family, friends, and community. Prioritizing important relationships provides us with support, companionship, and a sense of belonging amidst life's busyness.

Adapting to Change and Embracing Flexibility: Balancing work and leisure is a dynamic process that needs flexibility and adaptability. As our circumstances evolve, we stay open to new possibilities, adjusting our schedules and priorities with resilience and grace.

Appreciating the Joys of Life: Ultimately, finding balance is about embracing the sweetness of life—a celebration of joy, fulfillment, and the quest of happiness. It's about cherishing times of rest amidst our busy schedules and finding joy in everyday experiences. By fully embracing the richness of life, we respect the resilience and boundless potential of the human spirit.

CHAPTER EIGHT

FASHIONING TIMELESS STYLE

Fashion, a dynamic universe of ever-shifting trends and momentary vogues, offers as a stimulating canvas for expressing our distinct personalities and unleashing creative enthusiasm. However, amidst this maelstrom of alteration, there persists a magnetic allure—an essence of grace and sophistication that transcends the fleeting currents of time. Crafting timeless style is analogous to embarking on an exciting voyage—a journey that celebrates our originality, refines our tastes, and pays homage to the eternal allure of classical elegance.

Cherishing the Timeless Classics: At the root of timeless allure is a genuine admiration for the classics—those eternal silhouettes, textiles, and motifs that defy the passage of time. From the crisp proportions of a tailored jacket to the eternal flair of a little black dress, these timeless pieces form the cornerstone of sartorial elegance, providing a stage for personal expression and polished finesse.

Prioritizing Quality above Quantity: In a world overwhelmed with transient fads and disposable apparel, timeless style celebrates quality above quantity. It's about investing in beautifully created pieces that last the test of time—garments elegantly conceived, impeccably stitched, and fashioned from the finest materials. By embracing quality, we develop a wardrobe that transcends ephemeral fancies, expressing enduring grace and subtle allure.

Nurturing Personal Expression: Timeless style is an ode to individuality—a canvas where we paint the hues of our distinct personalities and artistic preferences. It's about constructing a wardrobe that matches our own likes, preferences, and character, allowing us to express ourselves authentically and with unflinching confidence. Whether through brilliant hues, bold accessories, or subtle nuances, timeless style celebrates the kaleidoscope of individual expression and revels in difference.

Embracing Versatility as a Virtue: Versatility lies at the heart of ageless elegance, providing the ability to smoothly move from dawn to twilight, season to season, and occasion to occasion. It's about investing in items that effortlessly adapt—garments as versatile as they are elegant, allowing for limitless permutations and combinations to fit our expanding lifestyles and discriminating sensibilities.

Championing Sustainability and Ethical Values: In the search of timeless style, sustainability and ethical fashion emerge as driving principles. It's about making deliberate decisions that minimize ecological footprint, preserve fair labor standards, and develop social responsibility. From picking for eco-conscious textiles to supporting ethical labels, timeless style becomes a testament to our values—a vow to cultivate a fashion industry that's sustainable, equitable, and conscientious.

Cultivating Confidence and Grace: Timeless style transcends just attire—it's an embodiment of attitude, thought, and demeanor. It's about establishing an aura of confidence, grace, and refinement that permeates every part of our life, transcending ephemeral trends and embracing the essence of real beauty.

Embracing the Journey of Self-Discovery: The quest of ageless style is a voyage—a journey of self-discovery, expression, and empowerment. It's about embracing our natural uniqueness, appreciating our originality, and embracing the various experiences that define our identity. In the fabric of ageless elegance, we unearth not just refinement and appeal, but also the profound beauty of honesty, tenacity, and inner fortitude.

As we navigate the kaleidoscope of fashion's ever-evolving terrain, let us embrace the art of constructing timeless style—a voyage that embraces the splendor of individuality, the attraction of classical elegance, and the enduring heritage of true refinement. From the precise lines of a tailored suit to the timeless charm of vintage accessories, timeless style begs us to explore, innovate, and relish in the everlasting elegance that characterizes us all.

EMBRACING PERSONAL STYLE EVOLUTION

Fashion surpasses mere apparel; it's a mirror reflecting our essence, our adventures, and our dreams. Personal style, ever-fluid, dances alongside our experiences, tastes, and perceptions. Embracing the growth of personal style is more than a nod to passing fads; it's a jubilee of originality, self-expression, and the beautiful trip of self-discovery.

Discovery Over Dictation: The evolution of personal style commences with self-exploration. It's about traveling varied aesthetics, experimenting with textures, hues, and forms, and providing ourselves the flexibility to build our individual fashion narrative. Instead of following closely to fashion principles, we pleasure in the excitement of exploration, enabling our curiosity to navigate new territories.

Evolving with Experience: Our personal style mimics the fabric of our life experiences—each encounter, triumph, and failure etches a significant imprint on our aesthetic sensibility. As we walk life's maze, our style transforms, echoing our metamorphosis, wisdom, and evolving viewpoints. Embracing personal style progression implies venerating the alchemy of experience and letting ourselves the ability to evolve organically.

Adapting to Change: Change is the heartbeat of life, and our personal style dances to its rhythm. Embracing personal style growth necessitates a readiness to adapt—to welcome novel trends, reject archaic preconceptions, and explore uncharted territories. It's about remaining receptive to change, greeting the unfamiliar with open arms, and providing oneself the opportunity to adapt, both in dress and spirit.

Expressing Individuality: Personal style is a dialect of self-expression—a canvas where we convey the hues of our persona, passions, and ideals. Embracing personal style growth is about exalting individuality, embracing the idiosyncrasies and intricacies that render us distinctive, and enabling our style to connect with the essence of our being, unapologetically.

Balancing Tradition and Innovation: Personal style progression is a delicate dance de deux between tradition and innovation—a fusion of timeless charm and current flair. It's about venerating ageless shapes and enduring pieces while infusing them with new flourishes and imaginative twists. Embracing personal style progression is an homage to history while embracing the infinite horizons of the future.

Celebrating Self-Expression: Personal style progression is a jubilee of self-expression—a monument to the kaleidoscope of our growing identities and the varied dimensions of our existence. It's about embracing the liberty to articulate ourselves genuinely, proudly, and audaciously, enabling our style to echo our innermost musings, ambitions, and dreams.

Embracing Uniqueness: In a world infatuated with conformity, embracing personal style progression is a declaration of our singularity, our individualism, and our intrinsic merit. It's about delighting in the fabric of difference, celebrating the numerous manifestations of style that enrich our lives, and realizing that true beauty rests not in conformity but in the mosaic of individuality.

As we embark on the adventure of personal style progression, let us revel in the miracle of self-discovery, the joy of exploration, and the transformative appeal of authenticity. Let us remember the riches of diversity, the boundless horizons of expression, and the profound appeal of expressing our real selves, one stylish stride at a time.

BEAUTY BEYOND AGE: SKINCARE AND FASHION TIPS

In a world enthralled by youth, the concept of beauty has often been linked with agelessness. However, true beauty respects no limitations of age. As we embrace the wisdom that comes with the passing of time, our approach to skincare and fashion evolves, revealing the keys of eternal allure. Here, we dig into the art of nourishing beauty beyond age, examining skincare and fashion suggestions that celebrate every stage of life.

Skincare Tips for Ageless Radiance:

Prioritize Hydration: Hydration is vital to retaining a young glow regardless of age. Invest on hydrating serums, moisturizers, and facial mists with nutrients like hyaluronic acid and glycerin to keep your skin supple and luminous.

Sun Protection Is Essential: Shielding your skin from the sun's harmful rays is necessary at any age. Incorporate broad-spectrum sunscreen into your regular skincare routine, and don't forget to reapply throughout the day, especially when spending time outside.

mild Cleansing Routine: Opt for mild cleansers that effectively remove pollutants without depleting your skin of its natural oils. Consider double cleansing to guarantee a thorough yet gentle removal of makeup and environmental contaminants.

Embrace Antioxidants: Antioxidants such as vitamin C and E help combat free radicals, which lead to accelerated aging. Incorporate antioxidant-rich serums and creams into your skincare regimen to protect and rejuvenate your skin.

Consistent Exfoliation: Regular exfoliation helps slough off dead skin cells, increasing cell turnover and revealing a new, bright complexion. Choose exfoliants suitable to your skin type, whether chemical or physical, and use them 1-2 times each week.

Fashion Tips for Timeless Style:

Invest in Quality Basics: Build your wardrobe around timeless classics such as well-fitted trousers, tailored blazers, and classic white shirts. Invest in high-quality pieces fashioned from sturdy fabrics that withstand the test of time.

Opt for Flattering Silhouettes: Embrace silhouettes that compliment your body form and accentuate your greatest features. Tailored shapes and structured clothes may create a professional and elegant image, regardless of age.

Play with Texture and Color: Experiment with textures and colors to give depth and intrigue to your clothing. Incorporate premium textiles like silk, cashmere, and linen into your wardrobe, and don't shy away from combining vivid hues and patterns to show your particular style.

Accessorize Thoughtfully: Accessories are the finishing touches that boost any ensemble. Invest in timeless accessories such as bold jewelry, classic handbags, and adaptable scarves that give flair and originality to your ensemble.

Confidence Is Key: Above all, display confidence in whatever you wear. Own your style choices with self-assurance and grace, appreciating the uniqueness that comes with age and experience.

ICONIC ROLE MODELS OF TIMELESS ELEGANCE

In a society typically dominated by transient fads and momentary celebrity, there exists a select handful of individuals whose essence transcends the passage of time. These lights, famed for their ageless elegance, serve as beacons of inspiration in an ever-changing landscape.

From the silver screen to the political stage, these iconic role models exemplify grace, poise, and sophistication in every part of their life. Their effect stretches well beyond mere aesthetics, going into the realms of culture, society, and human character.

Think of Audrey Hepburn, whose exquisite beauty and humanitarian initiatives continue to fascinate hearts decades after her departure. Her epitome of elegance wasn't just about fashion; it was a representation of her inherent love and compassion.

Consider elegance Kelly, whose move from Hollywood starlet to European queen embodied the marriage of glamour and elegance. Her ageless style and regal demeanor are an enduring icon of refinement.

Reflect on Cary Grant, whose suave charm and debonair manner established the standard for masculine grace. His exquisite taste in elegance and unshakeable charisma continue to inspire gentlemen worldwide.

Contemplate Jacqueline Kennedy Onassis, whose refined elegance and impeccable taste left an unforgettable imprint on the world of fashion and culture. Her signature ensembles and understated refinement continue to influence designers and tastemakers.

Ponder Katharine Hepburn, whose unusual attitude to style questioned standards and celebrated uniqueness. Her fondness for tailored suits and outspoken confidence opened the way for generations of women to embrace their uniqueness.

And let's not forget Fred Astaire, whose beautiful movements and faultless style characterized an era of elegance on the dance floor. His legacy serves as a reminder that true elegance rests not just in appearance, but in every step we take.

These iconic role models of ageless elegance remind us that true beauty transcends the surface and resonates on a deeper level. It's about expressing sincerity, integrity, and elegance in everything we do.

As we manage the difficulties of modern life, may we draw inspiration from these geniuses and seek to build our own sense of timeless beauty. For in doing so, we celebrate not only their legacies but the entire spirit of what it is to live with flair, substance, and refinement.

CHAPTER NINE

SPIRITUALITY AND INNER HARMONY

In the hectic modern world, when noise surrounds us and demands pull us in all ways, the quest for inner serenity and harmony becomes increasingly crucial. At the heart of this search lies spirituality, a deeply personal journey that transcends the tangible and links us to something higher than ourselves.

Understanding Spirituality:

Spirituality is the pursuit for meaning, purpose, and connection beyond the tangible realm. It encompasses a wide variety of beliefs, practices, and experiences, each unique to the individual traversing the path. While it may find expression in organized religion, spirituality stretches well beyond the bounds of religious theory, embracing many forms of faith, introspection, and transcendence.

Elements of Spiritual Practice:

Meditation and Mindfulness: Central to many spiritual traditions, meditation and mindfulness serve as doorways to inner serenity and awareness. Through peaceful thought and concentrated concentration, individuals acquire a greater awareness of themselves and their role in the cosmos.

Prayer and Contemplation: Whether through planned prayers or spontaneous communication with the divine, prayer serves as a conduit for connection and communion with the sacred. Contemplative techniques invite seekers to explore life's mysteries, struggle with existential problems, and find peace in moments of uncertainty.

Nature and Sacred Spaces: For many, nature acts as a sacred cathedral, encouraging reverence, awe, and renewal. Whether amidst towering woods, enormous deserts, or tranquil seas, the natural world generates a sense of interconnectedness and awe, anchoring us in the beauty of creation.

Service and Compassion: Spirituality finds expression not only in solitary thought but also in deeds of service and compassion towards others. Through unselfish generosity, kindness, and empathy, humans represent the concepts of love, unity, and social justice intrinsic to many spiritual traditions.

The Pursuit of Inner Harmony:

Inner harmony, the result of spiritual practice, is characterized by a profound sense of calm, balance, and alignment with one's actual self. It is the state of being in which the mind, body, and spirit resonate in perfect oneness, free from discord and disturbance. While the journey towards inner harmony may be long and riddled with challenges, its rewards are immeasurable—a life infused with purpose, resilience, and genuine joy.

NURTURING THE SOUL THROUGHOUT LIFE

Life, with its countless experiences and unfathomable mysteries, offers us an incredible opportunity for soulful discovery and growth. At the heart of our existence is the soul—a eternal energy that yearns for connection, purpose, and fulfillment. Nurturing the soul throughout life is not only a pursuit; it's a sacred journey of self-discovery, healing, and transformation.

The Essence of Soul Nurturing:

Cultivating Self-Awareness: To nourish the soul is to begin on a path of self-discovery. It begins with cultivating awareness—the willingness to examine the depths of our being, confront our fears, and embrace our vulnerabilities. Through introspection, meditation, and journaling, we unearth the truths that illuminate our path and form our destiny.

Embracing Authenticity: Authenticity resides at the core of spiritual life. It is the bravery to honor our beliefs, express our genuine selves, and live in alignment with our deepest convictions. By embracing authenticity, we liberate ourselves from the shackles of pretense and invite others to do the same, forging true connections and mutual understanding.

Seeking Meaning and Purpose: The quest for meaning and purpose enriches our lives with richness and depth. It motivates us to study the secrets of existence, pursue our passions, and contribute to the larger good. Whether via creative efforts, service to others, or spiritual practice, seeking meaning ignites the spark of inspiration that propels our journey.

Nourishing the Spirit: The soul lives on nourishment—nourishment of the body, mind, and spirit. It is discovered in times of calm, in communion with nature, in the laughter of loved ones, and in the embrace of community. Nourishing the spirit means honoring our need for rest, play, and rejuvenation, and emphasizing practices that restore our inner sources of strength and energy.

Embracing Transcendence: Transcendence urges us to rise above the constraints of ego and perception, to see the infinite expanse of consciousness that lies beyond. It is discovered in moments of amazement, wonder, and connection—moments that remind us of our oneness with all of creation. By accepting transcendence, we open ourselves to the endless possibilities that lie beyond the boundaries of the physical world.

The Journey Unfolds:

Nurturing the soul throughout life is not a goal to be achieved but a journey to be embraced—a journey defined by twists and turns, successes and tribulations, moments of joy and moments of grief. It is a trip that invites us to embrace the full range of human experience, to dance with the rhythms of life, and to enjoy the beauty of our shared humanity.

As we journey this sacred path, may we do so with open hearts and minds, with courage and compassion, knowing that each step we take gets us closer to the essence of who we are and the boundless possibilities that await us.

In feeding the soul, we acknowledge the divine spark that lies inside each of us—a spark that illuminates our path, guides our course, and reminds us that we are permanently united by the threads of love, grace, and eternal belonging.

Let us embrace this journey with reverence and gratitude, understanding that the greatest adventure of all is the journey back to ourselves.

Blessings on the path.

MEDITATION AND MINDFULNESS PRACTICES

In the frantic pace of modern life, amid the incessant buzz of external stimuli, lies a profound sanctuary—the practice of meditation and mindfulness. More than mere procedures, these practices offer a gateway to inner serenity, clarity, and profound transformation. Let us start on a journey inward, discovering the depths of meditation and mindfulness and their profound impact on our lives.

Understanding Meditation and Mindfulness:

Meditation is the technique of creating presence—a state of concentrated attention and awareness that transcends the oscillations of the mind. It invites us to anchor ourselves in the present now, to notice thoughts and sensations with non-judgmental awareness, and to build a sense of inner calm despite the bustle of daily life.

Mindfulness, on the other hand, is the discipline of bringing purposeful awareness to each moment, completely experiencing the richness of experience without attachment or aversion. It is about being totally present in whatever we do—whether eating, walking, or simply breathing—awakening to the beauty and wonder of life unfolding in real-time.

The Benefits of Meditation and Mindfulness:

Stress Reduction: Both meditation and mindfulness have been demonstrated to considerably reduce stress levels by activating the body's relaxation response, lowering cortisol levels, and generating a sense of inner peace and quiet.

Enhanced Emotional Well-being: By fostering awareness of our thoughts and emotions, meditation and mindfulness equip us to respond to life's obstacles with greater equanimity and resilience. They give a haven amidst the storms of the mind, enabling us to traverse the ups and downs of life with grace and presence.

Improved Concentration and Focus: Regular practice of meditation and mindfulness promotes cognitive function, increasing our capacity to concentrate, focus, and sustain attention on the work at hand. This heightened state of awareness translates into improved productivity, creativity, and clarity of thought.

Greater Self-awareness and Insight: Through introspection and self-reflection, meditation and mindfulness uncover the deeper layers of our psyche, illuminating patterns of thought, behavior, and belief that influence our perspective of reality. They invite us to explore the contours of our inner landscape, uncovering hidden truths and discoveries that lead to significant personal growth and transformation.

Cultivation of Compassion and Empathy: At the heart of meditation and mindfulness lies a deep sense of interconnectedness—a knowledge of our shared humanity and the inherent dignity of all beings. By growing compassion and empathy towards ourselves and others, we foster a more inclusive and peaceful environment, grounded in love, understanding, and acceptance.

Incorporating Meditation and Mindfulness into Daily Life:

Integrating meditation and mindfulness into our daily routines should not be frightening or hard. It can be as simple as taking a few moments each day to sit in stillness, examine the breath, or absorb the sensory pleasures unfolding around us. Whether through formal meditation sessions, mindful movement activities, or periods of quiet thought, the key rests in consistency, intention, and gentle perseverance.

EXPLORING SPIRITUAL DIMENSIONS OF AGING

As the fabric of life unfolds, each passing year draws us closer to the sacred threshold of aging—a journey marked by deep upheavals, challenges, and the soft embrace of spiritual growth. Beyond the physical changes that come with the passage of time, there is a deeper, more profound dimension: spiritual awakening, which invites us to investigate the essence of our being and the everlasting wisdom that exists inside.

Spiritual Dimensions of Aging:

Reflection and Contemplation: Aging asks us to pause and consider the tapestry of our lives—the pleasures, sufferings, victories, and tribulations that have molded our path thus far. It is a period for introspection, contemplation, and the development of wisdom gained through experience.

Embracing Impermanence: With each passing year, we are reminded of the fleeting aspect of life, which encourages us to treasure each moment, savor each breath, and appreciate the beauty of the present. Aging invites us to let go of our attachments to the past and future, and instead find peace in the everlasting dance of the present moment.

Cultivating Gratitude and Acceptance: As we age, we face the unavoidable reality of change—the shifting tides of our physical bodies, the evolution of our relationships, and the unraveling of life's mysteries. By embracing the spiritual components of aging, we cultivate thankfulness for the joys that abound while also accepting the realities that are beyond our control.

Deepening Spiritual relationship: As we age, we have the opportunity to deepen our relationship with the divine—to explore the sacred qualities of our existence and find peace in the divine presence within and around us. Whether via prayer, meditation, or acts of service, the spiritual path of aging invites us to surrender to the divine's guidance and trust in the unfolding of grace.

Finding Meaning and Purpose: As we approach the end of our lives, we are called to consider the legacy we want to leave behind—the impact we have had on the world and the people we have affected along the way. Aging encourages us to seek meaning and purpose in every moment, to live intentionally, and to embrace our humanity with grace and dignity.

Navigating The Spiritual Landscape:

Let us traverse the spiritual dimensions of aging with courage, grace, and an open heart. Let us approach the journey with humility and reverence, knowing that each step gets us closer to the essence of our being and the timeless mysteries that lie ahead.

Let us revere our elders' wisdom, whose presence enlightens the path with the light of experience and love. Let us appreciate the gift of each passing year, knowing that the embrace of aging contains the seeds of transformation and the prospect of spiritual regeneration.

In the sacred sanctuary of aging, may we find comfort in the divine whispers, strength in the depths of our souls, and the courage to embrace the fullness of life with joy and appreciation.

Blessings on your path through aging and spiritual development.

CHAPTER TEN

TECHNOLOGICAL INNOVATIONS FOR AGING WELL

In an era of rapid technological growth, the field of aging has not been left unaffected. From cutting-edge devices to new healthcare solutions, technology is changing the way we think about aging, allowing people to live more fulfilling, healthier, and independent lives. Let's look at the technological breakthroughs that are transforming the landscape of healthy aging.

1. Telehealth and Remote Monitoring: These platforms and gadgets are transforming healthcare delivery for older persons. From virtual doctor appointments to wearable sensors that measure vital signs, these technologies allow seniors to receive great care in the comfort of their own homes, decreasing the need for frequent hospital visits and improving overall well-being.

2. Smart Home Automation: Aging folks can benefit from smart home technology, which improves safety, convenience, and comfort. From voice-activated assistants to automated lighting and climate control systems, these advances allow seniors to keep their independence while being connected to the world around them

3. Wearable Health Trackers: Smartwatches and fitness bands offer real-time data on physical activity, heart rate,

sleep habits, and more. Monitoring important health measures enables older persons to take proactive efforts to improve their overall health and well-being, resulting in better results and a higher quality of life.

4. prescription Management Systems: Seniors with complex prescription regimens may struggle with managing their medications. Smart pill dispensers and medication reminder apps assist older folks in staying on track with their medications, ensuring they take the proper dose at the appropriate time and lowering the risk of adverse outcomes.

5. Social Connectivity Platforms: Older persons, especially those living alone or in care institutions, sometimes experience social isolation and loneliness. Social connectedness technologies, such as video chatting apps and online social networks, bridge the generation divide and allow seniors to maintain contact with family, friends, and communities, encouraging a sense of belonging and wellbeing.

6. Cognitive Health Technologies: Brain training applications and digital therapy programs are promising ways to maintain cognitive function and prevent age-related deterioration. These tools engage older persons in challenging tasks that test memory, attention, and problem-solving abilities, thereby increasing cognitive resilience and mental acuity.

7. Assistive Robotics: Assistive robotics are helping older persons navigate everyday duties and live independently. These technologies, ranging from robotic companions that

give social interaction and emotional support to robotic exoskeletons that aid in mobility and balance, enable seniors to keep their autonomy and dignity as they age.

ADVANCES IN HEALTHCARE TECHNOLOGY

In the ever-changing environment of healthcare, technology innovation is at the vanguard, driving transformative innovations that promise to redefine how we detect, treat, and prevent disease. From artificial intelligence to telemedicine, these game-changing advancements are altering the healthcare business and setting the way for an era of unrivaled efficiency, accessibility, and patient-centered care.

1. AI in Healthcare: AI has the potential to transform healthcare delivery by analyzing large volumes of data, recognizing trends, and offering actionable insights to assist clinical decision-making. AI-powered diagnostic technologies, predictive analytics, and personalized treatment algorithms have the potential to enhance patient outcomes, decrease medical errors, and maximize resource allocation in healthcare settings.

2. Telemedicine and Remote Monitoring: These technologies allow patients to receive healthcare services from home, removing geographical boundaries and increasing access to care. Telemedicine is changing the way patients and clinicians interact by enabling video consultations, virtual follow-ups, and wearable devices that

track vital signs, resulting in better convenience, efficiency, and continuity of care.

3. Robotics and Minimally Invasive Surgery: These techniques provide precision, flexibility, and quicker recovery times than traditional open surgery. Robotic-assisted devices allow surgeons to conduct complex surgeries with greater dexterity and precision, lowering the risk of complications while improving patient outcomes.

4. Digital Health and Wearable Devices: Digital health technology, such as wearables, smartphone apps, and remote monitoring tools, enable individuals to manage their health and wellness. These devices, which range from fitness trackers that monitor physical activity to smartwatches that track heart rate and sleep patterns, offer real-time insights into health data and support proactive health management.

5. Genome Sequencing and Precision health: Genome sequencing technologies are revealing the human genome's secrets, enabling personalized health techniques. By evaluating genetic variations and biomarkers, healthcare providers can tailor treatment plans, anticipate illness risk, and improve medication regimens, resulting in more targeted and effective therapy.

6. Virtual Reality (VR) and Healthcare Simulation: VR technology is transforming healthcare education and training by offering realistic, hands-on experiences for professionals. From surgical simulations to patient empathy training, virtual reality allows practitioners to develop their

abilities in a secure and controlled environment, increasing competency and improving patient safety.

7. Blockchain Technology and Health Data Security: Blockchain technology provides a safe and transparent framework for handling health data, assuring privacy, integrity, and interoperability amongst healthcare systems. Blockchain improves security by decentralizing data storage and offering cryptographic encryption, reducing the risk of data breaches and illegal access.

WEARABLE TECH AND AGING MONITORING

Wearable technology is a shining example of innovation in this age of technological wonders, transforming the way we track health and well-being, especially in older populations. Wearable technology, such as fitness trackers and smartwatches, provides a plethora of information and insights that enable people to take proactive measures to preserve their best possible health and vitality as they age.

1. Fitness Trackers: With the ability to monitor physical activity, heart rate, sleep patterns, and more in real time, fitness trackers are arguably the most popular type of wearable technology. These gadgets are incredibly useful for monitoring daily activity levels, establishing fitness objectives, and maintaining motivation to lead an active lifestyle in older persons.

2. Smartwatches with Health Monitoring Features: Smartwatches with health monitoring features, like blood oxygen saturation monitoring, heart rate sensors, and ECG (electrocardiogram) capabilities, offer thorough insights into cardiovascular health and general well-being. These gadgets allow for early intervention and preventive care by monitoring stress levels, detecting anomalies in heart rhythm, and even warning users of possible health issues.

3. Fall Detection and Emergency Response Systems: Elderly people and their carers can rest easy knowing that wearable technology is capable of both fall detection and emergency response. In the event of an accident or medical emergency, these gadgets use motion sensors and algorithms to detect falls and automatically notify emergency contacts or medical services. This ensures that help will arrive quickly.

4. Medication Reminder Devices: Wearable technology provides creative ways to guarantee dose compliance and medication adherence for senior citizens who are responsible for several prescriptions. By using alerts, notifications, and reminders to remind users to take their medications on time, smart pill dispensers and medication reminder devices lower the chance of medication errors and enhance treatment results.

5. Sleep Tracking Devices: These tools help older persons detect possible sleep problems and improve their sleep hygiene by offering insightful data on sleep patterns and quality. Through the monitoring of variables including sleep length, phases, and disturbances, these devices enable

users to make well-informed lifestyle decisions that facilitate revitalizing and peaceful sleep.

6. Activity Monitors for Cognitive Health: Wearable technology intended to track brain activity and cognitive health is a promising way to identify and treat age-related cognitive loss early on. These gadgets identify alterations in cognitive function and offer tailored interventions to promote brain health using cognitive evaluation tools, brainwave monitoring technologies, and machine learning algorithms.

7. Remote Health Monitoring Systems: These systems allow for the remote monitoring of chronic illnesses, post-acute care, and vital signs by combining wearable technology with cloud-based platforms and telehealth services. For older persons with chronic illnesses, these systems enable proactive treatment of medical conditions, lower hospital readmission rates, and enhance overall health outcomes.

THE DIGITAL WORLD'S ROLE IN STAYING YOUNG

In a world where the digital sphere is intertwined with our daily lives, the pursuit of youth takes on new meaning. From virtual exercise clubs to mindfulness apps and online learning platforms, the digital world provides an abundance of tools and resources to help people achieve vitality, resilience, and ageless living. Let's look at how the digital world is changing the paradigm of aging and empowering people to stay young in heart, mind, and spirit.

1. Fitness and Wellness applications: These applications provide easy access to exercise, diet, and mindfulness practices, empowering people of all ages to live better lifestyles from home. From personalized fitness regimens to meditation sessions and sleep tracking capabilities, these apps provide unique solutions to promote physical, mental, and emotional well-being.

2. Online Communities and Support Networks: The digital world fosters connections and communities beyond geographical boundaries, enabling virtual venues for individuals to discover companionship, support, and inspiration in their quest to ageless living. These platforms, ranging from social media groups to online forums and peer-to-peer networks, allow users to share their experiences, exchange ideas, and develop meaningful relationships with others who share their interests.

3. Online learning platforms promote lifelong learning and skill development, allowing individuals to pursue new interests and broaden their perspectives at any age. The digital world offers a multitude of educational opportunities to drive intellectual curiosity and personal growth across the lifespan, including language courses, art classes, coding workshops, and more.

4. Cognitive Fitness & Brain Training Games: Interactive exercises can improve cognitive skills, memory, and mental sharpness. From puzzles and quizzes to memory challenges and problem-solving exercises, these digital tools provide

enjoyable and practical ways to keep our brains healthy and active as we age.

5. Telehealth and Virtual Care Services: These platforms connect patients with healthcare practitioners, providing convenient access to medical consultations, preventive screenings, and chronic disease management from home. Telehealth enables individuals to take proactive efforts toward preventive health and well-being by utilizing technology to deliver individualized and patient-centered care.

6. The significance of digital detox and mindful computer use cannot be emphasized, especially in today's digital age. Digital mindfulness entails establishing boundaries, growing awareness, and prioritizing offline experiences that nourish the spirit and build genuine human connection. By establishing a balance between digital engagement and mindful presence, people may retake control over their relationship with technology and build a sense of inner peace and harmo**ny.**

CHAPTER ELEVEN

CELEBRATING UNCONVENTIONAL WISDOM

In a world dominated by conventional standards and established paradigms, there is a rich tapestry of unconventional wisdom—a richness of ideas, views, and techniques that question the status quo and push the frontiers of possibility. We may fully realize the potential of human creativity and collective wisdom by celebrating variety of view and embracing the spirit of innovation.

1. Diverse viewpoints: Unconventional knowledge relies on diverse viewpoints to enhance understanding of the world. It can be found in the voices of the marginalized, their experiences, and the perspectives of those who dare to challenge the dominant narrative. We build an inclusive, empathy-filled, and mutually respectful society by embracing multiple points of view and valuing the diversity of human experience.

2. Unconventional wisdom inspires creative problem-solving and innovation. It pushes us to think beyond the box, question assumptions, and investigate new possibilities. Whether in science, technology, the arts, or everyday life, unorthodox thinkers create innovations that change the world and influence history.

3. Embracing Failure and Resilience: Unconventional wisdom suggests viewing failure as a learning opportunity

and resilience as a source of strength. It serves as a reminder that difficulty frequently leads to growth, and that setbacks may be used to learn and grow. By establishing a mindset of resilience and perseverance, we may navigate life's obstacles with grace and resilience, coming out stronger and wiser.

4. Bridging Tradition and Innovation: Unconventional wisdom honors prior wisdom and embraces future possibilities. It understands that history serves as the foundation for progress, and that creativity thrives when it is based on a thorough understanding of cultural legacy and communal memory. By combining tradition and innovation, we create new paths forward while keeping the essence of what makes us human.

5. Fostering Authentic Connections: Unconventional wisdom promotes genuine connections that transcend superficial barriers such as race, gender, religion, and ideology. It acknowledges that true wisdom rests not in conformity, but in the bravery to be authentic and vulnerable. By building meaningful relationships based on trust, empathy, and mutual understanding, we may build communities that celebrate our shared humanity.

WISDOM VS. AGE: THE NUANCES

Passion projects are a powerful tool for personal growth, exploration, and self-discovery. They allow us to tap into our innate creativity, nurture lifelong learning, and embrace the spirit of exploration. These projects offer a platform for experimentation, innovation, and pushing the boundaries of what is possible. They also teach resilience and perseverance, enabling us to grow and evolve. Passion projects also provide a sense of purpose and meaning, connecting us with our deepest values and aspirations. They also foster connections and community, enriching our lives and nourishing our souls. The journey of passion projects is celebrated, not just the destination, as it celebrates the beauty of creativity, the joy of discovery, and the transformative power of following our hearts. As we embark on this journey, let us embrace the beauty of the creative process, the joy of exploration, and the fulfillment that comes from following our hearts

LEARNING FROM NON-TRADITIONAL SOURCES.

The pursuit of knowledge and personal growth often involves traditional education, textbooks, and academic institutions. However, the realm of wisdom extends beyond these boundaries, embracing a diverse array of non-traditional sources. Nature's classroom offers timeless wisdom on adaptation, interconnectedness, and the cyclical rhythms of existence. Personal experiences, indigenous wisdom, and artistic expression offer insights into sustainable living, community resilience, and harmonious coexistence with the natural world. Informal learning communities foster a culture of curiosity, innovation, and inclusivity, where individuals from diverse backgrounds come together to exchange ideas and co-create solutions to social and environmental challenges. The wisdom of elders and intergenerational dialogue offer guidance and perspective in navigating life's complexities. By honoring the wisdom of our elders and engaging in meaningful conversations across generations, we foster a culture of shared learning and interdependence that enriches our collective understanding of the world.

THE WISDOM OF EXPERIENCE AT ANY AGE

Wisdom is a timeless concept that emerges from the tapestry of life, encompassing both joyous and challenging experiences. It is crafted from the threads of our experiences, offering insights into the complexities of the human condition and the interconnectedness of all things. By embracing life's tapestry, we uncover hidden gems of wisdom within each moment, encounter, and choice we make. The power of perspective is also evident, shaping our understanding of the world. The wisdom gained through experience is not meant to be hoarded but to be shared generously, illuminating the path for future seekers of truth and understanding. It also teaches us resilience and adaptability, enabling us to navigate life's twists and turns with courage and grace. The wisdom of experience is a journey of self-discovery, awakening us to the beauty of our inner wisdom and the infinite possibilities that lie ahead.

CHAPTER TWELVE

PRACTICAL TIPS FOR EMBRACING AGELESSNESS

In the never-ending quest for understanding and enlightenment, the link between wisdom and age is a timeless conundrum, full of nuance and complexity. While age generally comes with experience, the development of wisdom goes beyond the passage of time, embracing a tapestry of life lessons, introspection, and personal growth. Let us delve into the complexities of this dynamic interplay, where the convergence of age and knowledge yields unique insights into the human experience.

Age is a concrete way to track the passage of time. It documents the milestones, successes, and trials that define our lives, providing glimpses into the ebb and flow of human existence. However, age does not guarantee wisdom; rather, it serves as the basis for wisdom to be grown and nurtured.

Wisdom is forged via experience, which comes from interactions with the world. It is the sum of our achievements and failures, pleasures and sufferings, loves and losses—a reservoir of knowledge and insight from which we draw lessons to better understand ourselves and others. Experience gives us perspective, empathy, and resilience, polishing the wisdom that comes from dealing with life's complexity.

Wisdom, unlike age or experience, goes beyond knowledge to embrace a deeper awareness of the human situation and interdependence. It stems from times of reflection, self-awareness, and thought in which we confront the facts that exist both within and without. Wisdom is the light that illuminates the route ahead, guiding us through the maze of existence with clarity, compassion, and discernment.

Cultivating Wisdom Across the Lifespan: Wisdom transcends age and circumstance. It is a lifelong journey of growth and discovery, punctuated by moments of joy, sadness, and transformation. Wisdom, whether young or old, invites us to embrace our entire humanity, learn from our mistakes, and seek for greater understanding and connection with ourselves and the world around us.

Honoring the Diversity of Paths: The journey to wisdom is as unique as the people who take it. Some may find knowledge in the peaceful contemplation of nature, while others may find it in the rush and bustle of city life. Some may gain insight from ancient books, while others may be inspired by elders' wisdom or children's innocence. Finally, wisdom has no fixed road or endpoint; it is a voyage of investigation, discovery, and self-discovery that unfolds differently for each person.

DAILY HABITS FOR TIMELESS LIVING

In the course of daily living, our habits shape the fabric of our existence, influencing our well-being, vitality, and sense of fulfillment. To live a life that transcends time, embrace timeless living as a conscious decision—a commitment to establishing everyday routines that nourish the body, mind, and spirit. Here are five transforming behaviors that will imbue your days with a sense of vibrancy and vitality:

1. Practice Morning Rituals of thankfulness: Begin each day with a ritual of thankfulness to set the tone for plenty and appreciation. Take a few seconds when you wake up to express thankfulness for the blessings in your life, such as the warmth of the sun, the air in your lungs, or the affection of family and friends. Develop a sense of amazement and admiration for the beauty around you, and take that thankfulness with you throughout the day.

2. Integrate mindful movement and exercise into your everyday routine to benefit your body and spirit. Find activities that make you happy and vital, whether it's a morning yoga practice, a brisk walk in nature, or a dance party in your living room. Pay attention to how your body feels, then move with intention, grace, and presence, respecting the sanctity of each movement.

3. Intentional Nutrition: Feed your body with wholesome foods that promote health and vigor. Accept full, plant-based foods high in minerals, vitamins, and antioxidants,

and enjoy each bite with attention and intention. Take the time to make meals with love and care, infused with appreciation and nourishment. Cultivate a mindful eating style by paying attention to your body's hunger and fullness cues and relishing each dish's flavors and textures.

4. Set aside time for introspection and stillness throughout the day to promote inner calm and clarity. Whether it's a peaceful meditation practice, a mindful breathing exercise, or a period of calm reflection, make time to connect with your inner wisdom and guidance. Allow yourself to calm down, breathe deeply, and focus on the rhythm of your breath and heartbeat to ground yourself in the present now.

5. Kindness and Compassion: Demonstrate kindness and compassion to yourself and others, cultivating a sense of connection and unity with all beings. Give a stranger a smile, aid a friend in need, or simply encourage and love yourself. Cultivate an open, generous, and loving heart, understanding that simple acts of kindness can have a ripple effect and influence the lives of many others.

6. Reflection and Gratitude Rituals: Enjoy moments of delight, growth, and learning as you wind down your day. Take a few moments to blog, meditate, or simply think on the events and lessons from your day. Express thankfulness for the obstacles that provided opportunities for growth, the friendships that developed, and the benefits that brought delight to your heart.

PLANNING FOR THE FUTURE WITH A YOUTHFUL MIND

The future is a tapestry of possibilities, ready to be stitched with threads of vision, ambition, and knowledge. While time brings changes and uncertainties, looking ahead with a youthful mind provides a transforming lens through which to traverse life's journey. Let's look at how embracing youthful vision and knowledge may illuminate the route ahead with vibrancy, purpose, and limitless possibilities.

1. Fostering Visionary Thinking: Adopt a visionary mindset as you plan for the future. Allow your mind to soar above the limitations of the present, visualizing alternatives that will rekindle your enthusiasm and creativity. Accept an attitude of inquiry and exploration, daring to dream large and pursuing those aspirations with persistence and enthusiasm.

2. Embracing Innovation and Adaptability: The future will be formed by technology, culture, and society, resulting in constant change and innovation. As you prepare for the future, embrace an innovative and adaptable spirit while keeping open to new ideas, opportunities, and possibilities. Cultivate a readiness to learn, grow, and change in response to changing circumstances, relying on resilience and flexibility to handle life's twists and turns.

3. Lifelong Learning: Embrace lifelong learning as a way to enrich your intellect, broaden your perspectives, and get a deeper grasp of the world. Seek for possibilities for

personal growth and development, whether through official education, self-study, or hands-on learning. Accept new challenges and experiences with curiosity and enthusiasm, knowing that every moment is an opportunity for growth and discovery.

4. Fostering Meaningful Connections: Connection and community improve the trip into the future, providing love, support, and friendship. Develop meaningful relationships with family, friends, mentors, and kindred spirits who will inspire and motivate you on your journey. Share your dreams, aspirations, and experiences with others, and be willing to accept advice, encouragement, and support in return.

5. Approaching the Future with Playfulness and Wonder: Embrace each day with youthful curiosity and joy. Find satisfaction in the basic joys of life, such as exploring nature, following creative hobbies, or participating in fun activities with loved ones. Cultivate a sense of amazement and awe for the beauty and magic that surrounds you, keeping your heart open to the limitless possibilities that lie ahead.

6. Living with Purpose and Intention: Align your activities and objectives with your deepest values to guide your future journey. Take some time to think about what is genuinely important to you and what provides you joy, fulfillment, and significance. Set significant objectives and dreams that speak to your heart and soul, and then take purposeful actions to bring them to life with courage, conviction, and dedication.

EMBRACING CHANGE AND FINDING JOY IN EVERY STAGE

Dear friends,

Life is a magnificent journey, with stages and transitions that form who we are and who we will become. These changes may appear frightening, even overwhelming at times, yet they contain tremendous potential for growth, discovery, and joy.

Accepting the inevitable changes in our lives is not enough; we must also embrace them with open arms and an open heart. It's about understanding that change is the very essence of life, a continual rhythm that pulls us ahead on our journey

Joy may be found at any stage of life, whether we are transitioning from adolescent to maturity, managing the intricacies of employment and relationships, or embracing the wisdom of our later years. Small moments of connection, whispers of inspiration, and triumphs of perseverance reveal the true richness of our lives.

Each stage has its own set of benefits and challenges, but they all provide opportunities to grow gratitude, resilience, and mindfulness. Embracing change allows us to discover our inner strength, deepest passions, and highest purpose.

So, while we navigate life's ever-changing landscape, remember to accept each stage with courage and grace. Let us celebrate the beauty of metamorphosis and the strength of regeneration. Above all, let us enjoy the voyage, understanding that each step brings new beginnings and limitless potential.

With love and thanks.

[james mason]